Beyond the Blueprint - Decoding the Elegance of Gene Expression

Edited by Morteza Seifi

Published in London, United Kingdom

Beyond the Blueprint - Decoding the Elegance of Gene Expression
http://dx.doi.org/10.5772/intechopen.1001795
Edited by Morteza Seifi

Contributors
Ahmed Kh. Abosalha, Bin Zhang, Chencheng Xu, Cristian-Radu Sisea, Garry A. Luke, Manda Venkata Sasidhar, Maria Emileva Krasteva, Martin D. Ryan, Paromita Islam, Sarwareddy Kartik Kumar, Satya Prakash, Shyam Mohapatra, Stephanie Makhlouf

First published in London, United Kingdom, 2024 by IntechOpen
IntechOpen is the global imprint of INTECHOPEN LIMITED, registered in England and Wales, registration number: 11086078, 167-169 Great Portland Street, London, W1W 5PF, United Kingdom

For EU product safety concerns: IN TECH d.o.o., Prolaz Marije Krucifikse Kozulić 3, 51000 Rijeka, Croatia, info@intechopen.com or visit our website at intechopen.com.

British Library Cataloguing-in-Publication Data
A catalogue record for this book is available from the British Library

Beyond the Blueprint - Decoding the Elegance of Gene Expression
Edited by Morteza Seifi
p. cm.

This title is part of the Genetics Book Series, Volume 4
Topic: Genomics
Series Editor: Kenji Ikehara
Topic Editor: Irina Vlasova-St. Louis

Print ISBN 978-0-85466-605-8
Online ISBN 978-0-85466-604-1
eBook (PDF) ISBN 978-0-85466-606-5
ISSN 3049-7094

IntechOpen Book Series

Genetics

Volume 4

Aims and Scope of the Series

"Genetics," which has been proud of its tradition since Mendel presented his research results in 1865, initially progressed quite slowly due to simple observational approaches of individuals and groups. However, the discovery of double-stranded DNA by Watson and Crick about 70 years ago triggered rapid progress in life sciences, including genetics, which was primarily conducted using Escherichia coli and bacteriophages infecting E. coli. Subsequently, genetics has achieved remarkable developments, such as understanding genetic disorders, including cancers, through research on the biogenesis and differentiation of plants and animals.
The two topics of this book series - Human Genetics, and Genomics - will address important areas of advancement in genetics.
Human Genetics: After fundamental genetics, initially studied with the main goal of revealing the functions of individual genes and proteins, genetics expanded from understanding the genetic system itself to understanding many infectious diseases caused by bacteria and viruses. Consequently, human beings are now overcoming infectious diseases by developing medicinal chemicals, including antibiotics and vaccines. However, genetic disorders remain challenging to cure up to now. Nevertheless, even the cure for them, including various cancers, is coming closer to reality due to the rapid progress of human genetics. In this way, the welfare of human life continues to improve, and even longevity, which was once a dream, has been achieved to some extent in recent years.
Genomics: On the other hand, the understanding of the comprehensive interrelationship of whole genes or whole proteins functioning in one organism has become possible now, as research has entered the era of genomics, owing to the rapid progress of base sequence analysis and bioinformatics. The development of genomics has further made it possible to understand the evolutionary processes of organisms through comparative studies among the genomes of many organisms.
This book series will discuss the findings obtained during the advancement of human genetics and genomics. It is also expected that this series will trigger the formation of a better world composed of human beings and all other organisms on Earth through discussions of research results obtained under the development of general genetics.

Meet the Series Editor

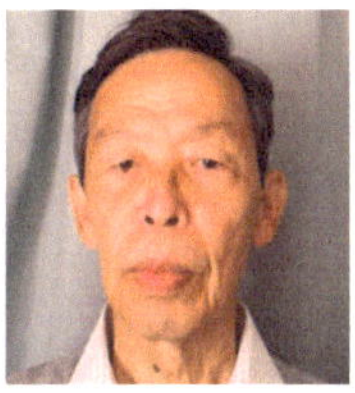

Kenji Ikehara graduated from the Department of Industrial Chemistry, Faculty of Engineering, Kyoto University in 1968. He received his B. Eng. (1968) and subsequently earned M. Eng. (1970) and D. Eng. (1976) degrees from Kyoto University. He began his career as a research associate in the Faculty of Science at the University of Tokyo before moving on to become an associate professor in the Faculty of Science at Nara Women's University. He was later promoted to professor and subsequently served as the dean of the Faculty of Science at Nara Women's University. Additionally, he held the position of director at the Nara Study Center of the Open University of Japan. For approximately 15 years, he focused his research on sporulation initiation of Bacillus subtilis. Later, he shifted his focus to the origins and evolutionary processes of microbial genes, the genetic code, proteins, and life. He has proposed several hypotheses, including the GC-NSF(a) hypothesis on the origin of genes, the GNC-SNS hypothesis on the genetic code, the protein 0th-order structure hypothesis on the origin of proteins, and the [GADV]-protein world hypothesis (GADV hypothesis) on the origin of life. Furthermore, he served as the local chair of the International Conference, Origin 2014, held in Nara in 2014.

Meet the Volume Editor

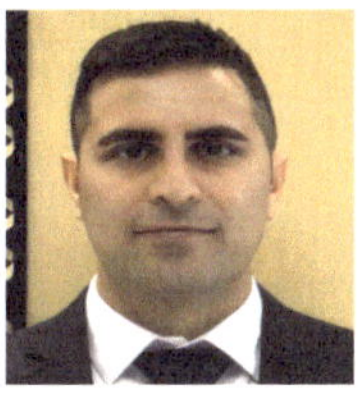

Dr. Morteza Seifi is an accomplished medical geneticist with a Ph.D. in Medical Genetics from the University of Alberta, Canada. He possesses extensive expertise in clinical genomics, variant interpretation, and bioinformatics, with his research featured in high-impact journals. Dr. Seifihas authored more than forty-six peer-reviewed publications and contributed to several books, with a primary focus on integrating innovative molecular and cytogenetic diagnostic techniques to advance personalized medicine. His dedication to education is demonstrated through his mentorship of the next generation of genomics professionals. Dr.Seifi's outstanding contributions to the field have earned him numerous accolades, including the prestigious Izaak Walton Killam Memorial Scholarship, one of Canada's largest and most prestigious endowment for Clinical and Translational Science activities.

Contents

Preface

The field of gene expression has witnessed remarkable advancements in recent years, with a growing understanding of the molecular mechanisms that govern how genes are regulated, expressed, and contribute to the complexity of life. *Beyond the Blueprint – Decoding the Elegance of Gene Expression* brings together contributions from leading experts, offering a comprehensive exploration of the latest research, techniques, and discoveries in this dynamic field.

This volume presents an in-depth examination of the various aspects of gene expression, from transcriptional regulation to posttranslational modifications, and how these processes impact cellular function, development, and disease. By exploring both well-established principles and emerging concepts, the book provides a broad understanding of gene expression's role in shaping biological systems.

A particular focus is given to the integration of innovative molecular diagnostic approaches, highlighting how these advancements are being applied in both research and clinical settings. The insights presented in this volume are expected to contribute to the ongoing efforts to uncover the mechanisms behind genetic disorders and develop targeted therapeutic strategies.

This edited volume is a valuable resource for researchers, clinicians, and students in molecular biology, genetics, and bioinformatics. By presenting a blend of foundational knowledge and cutting-edge research, the book aims to inspire further exploration and discovery in the realm of gene expression.

We extend our sincere gratitude to the contributors who have generously shared their knowledge and expertise. Their contributions have shaped this volume into a valuable reference for anyone interested in understanding the elegance and complexity of gene expression. We also wish to thank our colleagues, mentors, and institutions for their support throughout the editorial process.

We hope this volume will serve as a useful tool for readers seeking to deepen their understanding of gene expression and its far-reaching implications in science and medicine.

Morteza Seifi
University of Wisconsin-Madison,
Madison, USA

Chapter 1

Characteristics of Various Types of Plant Breeding

Cristian-Radu Sisea

Abstract

Plants have always been integral to human society and their (genetic) improvement has been carried out ever since humans became farmers. Breeders are seeking to alter plants in a permanent and heritable manner in order to enhance agricultural production relying on the scientific and technical advancements in molecular biology and biotechnology. Plant breeding simultaneously creates and exploits biological diversity (genetic variation), which are the main activities for plant breeders. Both plant domestication and traditional (conventional or classical) breeding depended on the natural processes and genetic potential of the species. However, innovations, such as mutation breeding, various biotechnological tools (*e.g. in vitro* techniques), and speed breeding, have been developed to enhance genetic gain and accelerate the breeding process. Furthermore, to improve selection, molecular markers were introduced. Strategies, such as molecular-assisted selection and genomic selection, are part of molecular (modern or nonconventional) breeding, which also includes two approaches based on genetic engineering: transgenesis and genome editing. The main characteristics of all these breeding tools — the essential assets for overcoming the agricultural challenges of modern civilization — and their relation to one another are presented in this chapter.

Keywords: traditional breeding, mutation breeding, speed breeding, molecular breeding, marker-assisted selection, genomic selection, transgenic breeding, genome editing

1. Introduction

Plants have always been, and still are, integral to human society because they provide food, feed, fiber, fuel, raw materials, medicines and other various bioactive compounds, esthetic pleasure, and solutions to various environmental issues. However, nearly all the plants that are useful today do not occur naturally but exist only because of human intervention that began thousands of years ago [1].

Early humans gathered what that they could find in the wild, but as their lifestyle changed from nomadic to sedentary, thousands of years ago, desirable plant species started to be selected and cultivated. This was the beginning of plant domestication [2], which represents the earliest form of plant breeding [3]. About 150 years ago, science revolutionized selection and breeding processes, facilitating and making them more efficient [4, 5]. To this day, plant traits and characteristics continue to be changed in order to better serve the needs of modern society [6]. The role of science and technology in plant breeding has increased continuously [4] and modern breeders rely on more and more sophisticated and efficient methods to create variability, discriminate among variants, and develop varieties (cultivars) for widespread cultivation [7].

The last five decades have been the most productive period in world agricultural history, saving billions of people from hunger and starvation [8]. The enhanced production has been based on overexploitation of natural resources and changing the natural environment, essentially entailing the modification of growing conditions [5, 8]. This was possible with the implementation of advanced agricultural technology, especially the application of production inputs such as fertilizers, irrigation, and pesticides [4, 5, 8]. However, this progress cannot cater to all the needs of mankind, and it will be even less sufficient in the coming years because of the increasing demands of human society [9]. So, for the future, the challenge is to ensure a sustainable rise in global agricultural production for a growing human population using finite natural resources and a shrinking agricultural land base due to industrialization, urbanization, and limiting factors, such as climatic or environmental changes [8–11]. In this context, the genetic improvement of crops is more important than ever.

In contrast to farmers, whose strategy is to enhance certain traits only temporarily — without tampering with the genetics of the organism — breeders seek to alter plants in a permanent and heritable manner so that genetic modifications are transmissible from one generation to the next [12]. The integration of newly developing technologies, such as molecular markers, OMICS, transgenesis, genome editing, and RNA interference into plant breeding, will provide the basic principles for developing modern breeding methodologies [4, 5, 13]. In this way, genetics coupled with other scientific knowledge (statistics, biometrics, biochemistry, bioinformatics, biotechnology, etc.) have the potential to overcome the aforementioned threats and challenges [8].

As an educator, I am concerned first and foremost with the students and the uninitiated, for whom understanding of all aspects of plant breeding is difficult to grasp, particularly because they are at the beginning of a challenging journey. As a result, it should be noted that this chapter is not intended for expert readers or an advanced audience as it will only offer a brief overview of the fascinating world of plant breeding, in order to provide up-to-date theoretical background and definitions. The main characteristics of the various types of plant breeding strategies are presented, starting with the fundamental principles of classical breeding and all the way to the advanced technologies of modern breeding, emphasizing approaches such as artificial induction of mutations, rapid generation advancement, the use of molecular markers, transgenesis, and genomic editing.

2. Plant breeding

It should be noted that the terms plant breeding and plant improvement are used synonymously [5]. One of the best-suited definitions for plant breeding is the one given by [12]: "the art and science of improving the heredity of plants for the benefit of humankind." Other definitions emphasize the changing, altering, or manipulation of genetic patterns, genetic make-up, genetic information, genome, or genetics of plants in order to produce desired traits or characteristics, to increase their value, or to make them a better fit for human purposes. Basically, the plant breeding process encompasses techniques for producing, selecting, and fixing superior plant phenotypes in order to develop new, improved cultivars that better meet the requirements of farmers and consumers [14, 15].

Many authors state that the scientific basis for plant breeding was established by the ground-breaking work of Gregor Johann Mendel in the middle of the nineteenth century. However, the principles put forth by Charles Darwin and Alfred Russell Wallace during the same period are equally important since breeding is nothing less than a particular form of evolution. At the beginning of the twenty-first century, the science of crop improvement is being transformed once again by molecular breeding, which integrates the latest breakthroughs in biological research — namely molecular biology and biotechnology — with traditional breeding practices [15–19]. As science and technology advance, modern breeders are able to make their activities more and more predictable and precise, with plant breeding becoming indispensable to modern human society [20]. Thus, the development of a new crop variety is an example of agricultural biotechnology that includes both traditional breeding techniques and modern methods [1, 21], such as molecular markers and genetic engineering.

As mentioned before, plant breeding is often likened to evolution [5]. Yet, a crucial distinction between the two is that evolution is a natural and extremely slow process, whereas plant breeding is a relatively quick artificial one [2]. Moreover, natural evolution increases the fitness of the populations or species, whereas plant breeders aim to direct the population toward specific and predetermined goals — often related to yield, nutritional value or other commercial traits — that are generally not concerned with fitness because modern farmers can grow plants under artificial conditions [5]. It should be noted, however, that in recent years, there has been a shift toward improving adaptability to abiotic or biotic stress factors in order to make better use of land resources while also taking climate change into consideration [22].

The development of new cultivars entails two basic activities: assembling genetic variability and discriminating among variants — selection — in order to identify and advance desirable genotypes (individuals) that meet the breeding objectives [7]. These two stages are followed by the evaluation and release of the cultivar [5].

Depending on the approaches and techniques employed by breeders, which keep evolving along with science and technology, there are two basic categories of plant improvement: traditional (conventional) and molecular (nonconventional) [4, 20]. These two categories and their characteristics will be presented in the remainder of this chapter.

3. Traditional plant breeding based on selective breeding

Traditional plant breeding, also called classical or conventional breeding, is the development of crop varieties by using natural processes and conservative, older, simpler, and relatively low-tech tools to modify an organism's genetic information within the natural boundaries of its species [1, 5]. The absence of modern developments or lack in sophistication is not implied here as traditional breeding entails both basic and advanced methods [23]. In fact, practices used in traditional breeding may include features of biotechnology such as tissue and cell culture, protoplast fusion techniques for somatic hybridization, techniques for embryo rescue to overcome incompatibility barriers, advanced pollination procedures and *in vitro* fertilization, techniques for polyploidization a haploidization, and mutation breeding [4, 14, 23]. However, the fundamental method remains modification through selective breeding [1, 14], also called artificial or phenotypic selection, which is based on phenotype evaluation for identifying individuals with desirable traits [3, 5, 24]. Consequently, the methods and techniques used by conventional breeders rely heavily on the species' mode of reproduction — self-pollination, cross-pollination, or clonal (vegetative) propagation — and contrast with the newer and more innovative breeding tools of molecular breeding [5]. This is why, the initial statement is defining the traditional breeding approach by actually comparing it to the most cutting-edge breeding technologies. In much the same manner, EU legislation on genetically modified (GM) organisms (GMOs) — *that is.* Directive 2001/18/EC — clearly delineated traditional breeding from what was, at the time, the most innovative methodology for crop improvement — transgenesis or recombinant DNA technology [23]. This idea was rightly extended to include other genetic engineering tools – *that is.* genome editing — which are considered to have revolutionized crop improvement and biological research and which will be presented in Subchapter 4.2.2. In conclusion, all genetic engineering methods that enable the creation and introduction of novel variation into genomes through genetic engineering should be separated from traditional breeding [25]. This is especially true from a technical point of view, but the legal implications are more nuanced; these will be discussed further in Subchapter 4.2.2.

Artificial selection can be performed on naturally occurring individuals, but, more often, on offspring resulted from controlled crosses, also called matings or hybridizations. Therefore, in conventional breeding, desirable traits are assembled into a new cultivar from different but very closely related plants — usually belonging to the same species [4]. As such, the individuals resulting from conventional breeding only display characteristics already present in the genetic potential of their species because new genes (and characteristics) are not introduced [5]. Also, when none of the individuals on which selection is performed possesses a certain gene variant controlling a particular trait, it is not possible to select that specific trait [1].

It should also be noted that in a controlled mating all of the genetic material between the two individuals being bred, which could mean tens of thousands of genes (maize, for example, has approximately 32,000 genes), is shuffled. The results of such a mix can be very unpredictable because of the large number of combinations — *that is.* genotypes or individuals — it can generate and finding the best one could be very difficult [1].

Artificial selection is the oldest technique for crop improvement and still remains widely used [20, 26]. This has actually been the main process through which, over the years, humans have gradually and systematically favored traits that have increased the utility of plants [1, 5].

3.1 Mutation breeding

Plant breeding relies on genetic variation — "heritable variation is the lifeblood of plant breeding" [5] — for selecting desired genotypes or traits [27–29].

In nature, mutations — the heritable changes to an individual's genetic makeup [14, 30] — represent one of the essential mechanisms for genetic variation and evolution — individuals with a novel trait may be preferentially selected because of their superior fitness determined by the novel (mutant) adaptive features [28, 29, 31]. Mutations are in fact the new gene variants (alleles) controlling new traits that are passed on from parents to offspring [28–30].

Humans have used natural genetic variation since they started cultivating plants by actually (and also unknowingly) selecting for the alleles that were beneficial and suitable to their needs [9]. The natural rate of mutation is nevertheless very low and insufficient for generating all the variation that breeders would like to have for their breeding programs [26], which have to run at a much faster pace than natural evolution. To overcome this limitation, plant breeders can artificially induce additional mutations by using physical (*i.e.* different types of high-energy radiation) or chemical (*e.g.* ethyl methanesulfonate and dimethyl sulfate) mutation-causing agents – mutagens [28–30, 32, 33]. This way of generating new variation to be exploited in the breeding process is called mutation breeding. Consequently, the genetic variation used in plant breeding could be: (1) found in the natural, existing gene pool; (2) obtained through crossings (hybridizations) that shuffle existing variation into new combinations without creating novel gene variants; and (3) the result of artificial mutagenesis which actually means generating new alleles.

Usually, mutation breeding is considered part of conventional or traditional breeding [23, 28–30, 32, 33], but different opinions can be found as well:

- "Genetic transformation and mutation breeding, as nonconventional breeding tools for plant improvement, are outlined and selection *in vitro* against a fungal toxin isolated from *Mycosphaerella fijiensis* is presented in more detail." [34];

- "... nonconventional breeding of banana, more specifically genetic transformation, protoplast culture, somatic hybridization and EMS-induced mutation ..." [35].

EU legislation on GMOs — *that is.* Article 3(1), in conjunction with Annex I B of Directive 2001/18/EC — is very clear on this topic: mutagenesis — introducing variations in the plant genome using radiation or chemicals — is regarded as traditional breeding and is explicitly exempt from the scope of the Directive 2001/18/EC, on the basis that it has a long history of safe use [23, 32, 33, 36].

With more than 3000 mutant crop varieties in more than 200 plant species having been officially released worldwide [28, 29, 31, 37], mutation breeding continues to be an important tool for today's plant improvement efforts together with the more advanced and precise nonconventional techniques [28, 29, 31].

3.2 Speed breeding

Several years are required for developing cultivars using conventional procedures for generation advancement (to the next breeding cycle). In order to achieve a rapid generation advancement (RGA) — *that is.* the shortening of breeding cycles — with more than three to four generations per year, a relatively unsophisticated and highly adaptable platform for plant cultivation was perfected [38–42]. Research on this topic had been reported as far back as 1880 [39, 41], based on the idea of growing plants under artificial light that was experimented with by botanists [40, 41]. The RGA approach was first proposed just before World War 2, then modified in the 1960s, and its most recent form — speed breeding — was introduced only a few years ago [39, 42].

Just like mutation breeding and molecular breeding (Subchapter 4), speed breeding is aimed at accelerating genetic gain [38–40]. For this, plants are cultivated under fully enclosed environmental conditions, in growth chambers or greenhouses, where crop-specific optimal light (quality, intensity, and duration), temperature, and humidity can be artificially controlled [30, 38–40, 42].

The basic and simple procedures of speed breeding can be easily adopted. However, this approach is much more effective in enhancing genetic gain when integrated with other modern strategies [39]. To produce greatly improved outcomes, speed breeding can be combined with:

- marker-assisted selection [38]; marker-assisted selection is presented in Subchapter 4.1.1;
- high-throughput genotyping — *that is.* genomics-assisted breeding — combination that represents the most effective strategy for quick variety development [40]; genomics-assisted breeding is presented in Subchapter 4.1.2;
- genome editing techniques [11, 40], an approach called *express edit* [40]; genome editing is presented in Subchapter 4.2.2;
- automated or high-throughput phenotyping [40, 42].

This type of accelerated plant breeding reduces the time, space, and manpower needed to advance plant generations more rapidly and develop varieties at a quicker pace, so speed breeding was adopted worldwide, with already well-established protocols in many important staple crops [38–42].

4. Molecular plant breeding

The agricultural challenges of modern society, determined by population growth, climate change, limited resources, and the constraints of conventional breeding, require increasingly innovative, modern methodologies to be applied for the genetic improvement of crops [17, 43, 44]. In the past few decades, due to the progress in science and technology — *that is.* the considerable increase of knowledge on genes and their function at the molecular level — advanced, new tools for plant breeding have been added to those that have been in use for a long time — *that is.* traditional breeding [8, 42]. The various umbrella terms describing these new, advanced breeding methods are nonconventional (or unconventional), modern, and molecular. Molecular breeding is arguably the most appropriate and commonly used of the aforementioned terms. The following are some straightforward definitions for molecular breeding:

- "Application of molecular biology in plant breeding is molecular breeding." [3].
- "Similarly, the recent integration of advances in biotechnology, genomic research, and molecular marker applications with conventional plant breeding practices has created the foundation for molecular plant breeding, an interdisciplinary science that is revolutionizing twenty-first century crop improvement." [15].
- "Recent progress in biotechnology and genomics has expanded the breeders' horizon providing a molecular platform on the traditional plant breeding, which is now known as plant molecular breeding." [16].
- "Molecular breeding applies molecular biology tools to accelerate the breeding process." [17].

- "Molecular breeding is a modern technique that refers to the combined application of plant biotechnology and breeding for crop improvement." [18].

- "Modern plant breeding techniques came into being when molecular techniques were integrated along with conventional breeding techniques in order to achieve higher genetic gains." [19].

Taking into consideration the primary components of molecular breeding outlined in the previous definitions — *that is.* molecular biology, biotechnology, molecular markers, and genomics — it can be concluded that its essential tools are molecular biology techniques. For better understanding what the concept of molecular breeding entails it is necessary to consider other, more detailed opinions on this topic, which are quite heterogeneous. This is due in part to the fact that terms such as genetic engineering, biotechnology, and molecular marker, used to describe molecular breeding are, in their turn, not always agreed upon by all authors.

Most often, molecular breeding encompasses the use of molecular markers and genetic engineering, as shown by the following definitions:

- "The areas of molecular breeding include QTL [quantitative trait locus] mapping or gene discovery, marker-assisted selection and genomic selection, genetic engineering, and genetic transformation." [3]; here, it should be noted that genetic transformation is not included in genetic engineering.

- "To this end, recent advances in transcriptome profiling, functional genomics, proteomics, and metabolomics approaches, coupled with molecular marker-assisted breeding and transgenic technology have made significant contributions in enhancing the efficiency of cotton breeding; these methods are collectively referred as molecular breeding." [45]; here, the authors do omitted genome editing; this also applies to the next definition.

- "Molecular breeding in cotton includes traditional cotton breeding supplemented with marker-assisted breeding using advances in molecular-marker technology and QTL mapping (which includes marker-assisted backcrossing and marker-assisted recurrent selection), genomics (known as genomics-assisted breeding), and transgenics technology." [45];

- "Therefore, combination of conventional and modern breeding approaches, such as backcrossing, foreground and background selection, phenotyping, gene pyramiding, marker-assisted selections, identification of quantitative trait loci, and many more can be used to have new and improved varieties. Further, biotechnological approaches such as identification of genes by using markers, genetic transformation, regulating signal transductions, and different omics approaches (genomics, transcriptomics, proteomics, and metabolomics) are choice of scientists to develop next generation crops to tackle the challenge of having sustainable agriculture, adverse effect of climate change, and to feed the looming population." [46].

- "Molecular breeding may be defined in a broad sense as the use of genetic manipulation performed at DNA molecular levels to improve characters of interest in plants and animals, including genetic engineering or gene manipulation, molecular marker-assisted selection, genomic selection, etc." [47].

There are instances when the authors reference only one of the elements mentioned above, either molecular markers or genetic engineering:

- "Molecular breeding is used to describe several modern breeding strategies, including marker-assisted selection, marker-assisted backcrossing, marker-assisted recurrent selection and genome-wide selection or genomic selection." [3].
- "DNA markers are also called molecular markers in many cases play a major role in molecular breeding." [47, 48].
- "Marker-assisted or marker-based backcrossing is regarded as the simplest form of marker-assisted selection, and it is the most widely and successfully used method in practical molecular breeding." [47, 48].
- "The use of DNA markers in plant breeding is called marker-assisted selection and is a component of the new discipline of "molecular breeding." [49].
- "The classical approach for molecular breeding is heavily dependent on marker-assisted selection and the trait linked DNA markers as an alternative to support phenotypic screening." [50].
- "Molecular breeding uses molecular biology tools in breeding crop plant. It includes approaches such as marker-assisted selection and qualitative trait loci mapping." [51].
- "Single and multigene transgenesis is the current strategy since the past one decade, which if aptly exercised alongside other molecular breeding strategies, can yield satisfactorily performing drought tolerant crop plants." [52].

Other authors present molecular breeding as pertaining either to molecular markers or genetic engineering:

- "Molecular breeding is the DNA marker-assisted breeding that calls for sophisticated instrumentation and facilities." [3].
- "Molecular breeding, or MAS, refers to the technique of using DNA markers that are tightly linked to phenotypic traits to assist in a selection scheme for a particular breeding objective." [53]
- "Molecular breeding approaches target on specific regions on the DNA and therefore are called as marker-assisted breeding. This is often taken from QTL mapping of the quantitative trait. MAB involves numerous modern plant breeding strategies, comprising marker-assisted selection, marker-assisted backcrossing, marker-assisted recurrent selection, and genome-wide selection or genomic selection. Marker-assisted selection (MAS) is a breeding approach that involves integration of detection and selection of DNA marker with a conventional breeding program." [54].
- "Called molecular plant breeding, plant breeders may now access genes from the animal kingdom for plant improvement, but not without controversy." [5].

Sometimes molecular breeding — potentially referring to molecular markers — and genetic engineering are seen as two different components of modern breeding methods:

- "The final part has an excellent discussion of advanced techniques of plant breeding, such as tissue culture, genetic engineering, molecular breeding, and application of genomics." [3].
- "Molecular breeding and [genetic engineering] also have benefits over conventional breeding because they make it tranquil to grow crops with many nutritional traits of interest." [18].
- "Now, new innovative additional plant breeding tools, including molecular breeding and plant biotechnology, are available to plant breeders, which have a great potential to be used along with the conventional breeding methods for sustainable agriculture." [55]; here, plant biotechnology most probably refers to genetic engineering.
- "For introduction of desirable traits molecular breeding and transformation technique have also been used widely." [56].

Certainly, there are many other particular definitions for molecular breeding, its components, and the relations between them.

Conventional techniques are time-consuming, so one of the most important advantages of molecular breeding is the possibility of reducing the duration of the crop development process by years [18]. However, due to its complexity, the successful application of molecular breeding requires sophisticated, high-tech infrastructure and deep knowledge and specialization [44].

4.1 Molecular markers in plant breeding

While significant genetic improvements have been achieved using classical breeding methods — based on phenotypic selection [3, 24] — the employment of molecular biology and genomics tools — *that is,* molecular or DNA markers — has the potential to enhance genetic gains even more by making selection easier, faster, and more accurate, which will reduce the generation interval and the costs and will improve the overall speed and efficiency of the breeding process [57–59]. An important advantage of using molecular markers is that genotypic evaluation can be done off-season and the influence of the environment is negligible [60]. Therefore, in recent decades, the focus shifted from phenotype-based to genotype-based selection [3], making molecular markers one of the main components of modern breeding. The two primary types of molecular marker-based strategies used in plant breeding are presented in the following subchapters.

4.1.1 Marker-assisted selection and breeding

Marker-assisted or marker-aided selection (MAS) is the selection of individuals with desirable traits based on the direct analysis of their genetic makeup (genotype) and it can be employed alone or in combination with classical methods [57]. Marker-assisted breeding (MAB) includes several molecular analysis-based applications intended to enhance mating designs, genetic testing and screening, deployment strategies and overall quality control in plant improvement programs [57].

Only a few general aspects are addressed here, while the various types of molecular markers with their features, advantages and drawbacks will not be discussed. These general aspects, that specialists have different views on, are related to how the concept of molecular markers should be perceived. One such issue is the influence of the molecular marker on the target characteristic. In the following examples MAS is presented as a form of indirect selection — the assumption that the marker closely associates with one or more genes of interest, due to genetic linkage, but does not influence the target characteristic:

- "Marker-assisted selection or marker-aided selection (MAS) is a process whereby a marker (morphological, biochemical or one based on DNA/RNA variation) is used for indirect selection of a genetic determinant or determinants of a trait of interest (*i.e.* productivity, disease resistance, abiotic stress tolerance and/or quality)." [3].

- "One of the most important methods of molecular breeding is MAS, the use of DNA markers that are tightly linked to target loci as a substitute to assist phenotypic screening." [17].

- "MAS is an indirect selection process, where individuals for a particular trait of interest are selected based on the known markers linked to it." [24].

- "MAS is the process of using morphological, biochemical, or DNA markers as indirect selection criteria for selecting agriculturally important traits in crop breeding." [61].

- "Marker-assisted selection is a strategy to accelerate genetic gain in conventional breeding programes by selecting plants with a desirable combination of genes using tightly linked markers." [62].

However, indirect selection is only one type of MAS, direct selection being also possible:

- "All forms of indirect selection involve selection for one trait to make improvement in a different trait, called the target trait. A second and developing, form of MAS is to select directly on the individual alleles at one or more loci affecting polygenic traits. This form of marker-assisted selection requires knowledge, at the molecular level, of some or all of the genes controlling the target trait and can be viewed as direct selection, rather than indirect selection, since selection is for specific, favorable alleles at those loci." [57].

- "Marker-assisted selection is a newly emerging approach due to which various problems of conventional breeding avoid and enhance the selection criteria of phenotypes with the selection of genes, either indirectly or directly." [63].

- "Molecular genetic analyses of quantitative traits lead to the identification of two broadly different types of genetic loci that can be used to enhance genetic improvement programes: causal mutations and presumed non-functional genetic markers that are linked to QTL (indirect markers). [...] Whereas causative polymorphisms give direct information about genotype for the QTL, the use of indirect markers for QTL mapping and for selection is based on the existence of linkage disequilibrium (LD) between the marker and the QTL" [64].

- "Secondly, some SNPs [*single nucleotide polymorphism*] are located in coding regions and directly affect protein function. These SNPs may be directly responsible for some of the variations among individuals in important traits." [65].

It is also important to understand that molecular markers represent just one of the several types of markers that can be used in plant breeding. The classification of markers can vary, but the concept is rather consistent:

- "Genetic markers used in genetics and plant breeding can be classified into two categories: classical markers and DNA markers. Classical markers include morphological markers, cytological markers and biochemical markers." [47].

- "Such variations occurring at different levels, *that is.* at the morphological, chromosomal, biochemical, or DNA level can serve as the genetic markers." [66].

- "Genetic markers are classified: based on visually evaluated traits (morphological and productive traits), based on gene product (biochemical markers), and founded on DNA analysis (molecular markers)." [67].

Usually, genetic markers encompass all of the other types of markers and can be defined as:

- "... the biological features that are determined by allelic forms of genes or genetic loci and can be transmitted from one generation to another, and thus they can be used as experimental probes or tags to keep track of an individual, a tissue, a cell, a nucleus, a chromosome or a gene." [47];

- "... any stable and inherited variation that can be measured or detected by a suitable method, and can be used subsequently to detect the presence of a specific genotype or phenotype ..." [66]; this definition emphasizes only indirect selection;

- "... a broad term for any visible or assayable phenotype or the genetic basis for assessing of the observed phenotypic variability." [67].

The definition of molecular markers also varies between authors, especially when considering different fields of study and no attempt will be made here to reconcile them. Below are some appropriate definitions for molecular markers applicable to plant breeding:

- "The markers revealing variations at the DNA level are referred to as the molecular markers." [66].

- "Molecular marker is a term used to refer to a specific DNA variation between individuals that has been found to be associated with certain characteristics." [67].
- "A molecular or DNA marker is the difference in DNA nucleotide sequence — between individual organisms or species — that is in proximity or tightly linked to a target gene that expresses a trait." [68]; it should be noted that the authors emphasize only indirect selection.

MAS is probably both the least sophisticated and the most widely used approach in practical molecular breeding because of its simplicity, especially when compared to the other molecular breeding strategies.

4.1.2 Genomic selection and genomics-assisted breeding

MAS has demonstrated its practicality and feasibility in the enhancement of qualitative traits — features associated with one or very few major genes — but its usefulness in improving quantitative traits — polygenic traits controlled by hundreds or thousands of minor genes, with small effects — is limited [24, 69]. To address this issue, a powerful new approach called genomic selection (GS) or genome-wide selection (GWS) was developed [24]. This new approach became feasible only with the development of new generations of DNA sequencing technologies that revolutionized biological research and genomics by drastically reducing the costs and duration of sequencing [59]. High-throughput genotyping enables the routine implementation of GS to fully benefit crop improvement [59].

Without prior knowledge of relevant QTLs or other molecular markers [69], GS uses dense single SNPs distributed across the whole genome to estimate the genetic merit of individuals of a breeding population and to facilitate the selection of candidates for the next breeding cycle [24, 69, 70]. GS shows great potential for resolving the issue of selection of traits associated with multiple genes [71] because it can theoretically account for the effect, no matter how small, of every piece of genetic information — gene or otherwise — from a genome [72], for which conventional selection and MAS are difficult and time-consuming to apply [71]. Therefore, GS ensures high accuracy and allows for a substantial reduction in the duration of the breeding cycle, while also decreasing the costs associated with extensive phenotyping, and thus accelerating genetic gains and improving the overall efficiency of the breeding process [60, 73].

The possibility of analyzing individuals through whole genome sequencing has turned GS and other genomics-assisted breeding (GAB) tools into powerful assets [3, 60, 72], which enable the integration of genomics with conventional phenotyping in order to facilitate the prediction of phenotype from genotype [3, 60]. In this context, the breeder can make a comprehensive characterization of the genetic variation in order to find the best alleles — *that is.* to accumulate beneficial alleles and purge deleterious ones [11] — and combinations of alleles (haplotypes) for future crop cultivars [3, 11, 60].

Implementation of GS requires that individuals in a fully phenotyped population v generally called training population — are genotyped using genome-wide markers instead of selected molecular markers. Available phenotypic and genotypic information is employed to build a statistical predictive model that estimates the breeding values of the alternative alleles of all the markers. The additive sum of all marker effects is used to calculate the genetic merit of each individual and the genomic estimated breeding value (GEBV) of the training population. GEBV can then be utilized to estimate the phenotypic value of individuals in a breeding program employing solely their genotypic data. In this regard, the selection of individuals in subsequent generations is based purely on GEBVs. This general outline of the genomic selection process is based on information published by [11, 24, 59, 60, 70, 72, 73].

However, there are certain factors that may influence the accuracy of the genomic prediction: the size and genetic diversity of the training and breeding populations, as well as the genetic relationship between the two, the heritability of the target trait, the influence of the environment on the initial population, the density of markers, the choice of statistical models used to estimate breeding values, and the accuracy of the phenotyping [24, 69, 72].

In conclusion, there is great potential in GS and GAB, and overcoming the limitations these technologies are currently facing will make their routine implementation possible in plant breeding [24, 72, 74], which might lead to replacing phenotypic selection and MAS, at least in the analysis of complex traits [59].

4.2 Genetic engineering in plant breeding

Due to its most defining attribute — the possibility of direct and highly accurate manipulation of genetic information — genetic engineering (GE) has transformed both the way in which biological studies are performed, by becoming an essential tool for understanding the genetic basis of biological processes and the possibilities of applying acquired knowledge [9, 75, 76]. The manipulation of genetic material is intended to induce gene function-level changes — gene inactivation, overexpression of an already existing (native) gene, or synthesis of a new compound and integration of a new function after the insertion of a new gene — that will, in turn, alter the phenotype. Thus, GE has found numerous applications in all the main sectors of human activity — industry, medicine, and agriculture — including plant breeding.

GE represents the foremost biotechnological approach that is used in modern breeding for the genetic improvement of crops, with two basic components: transgenesis or transgenic technology and genome or gene editing [77]. Both of them allow twenty-first-century breeders to alter the genome of an organism and to create new heritable variability through the direct manipulation of the genes controlling the traits of interest [16]. There is, however, an essential difference between the two: the origin of the manipulated genetic material.

In the case of transgenesis, genetic material from two (or more) species is used — *that is.* combined. Basically, the transfer of genetic material — *that is.* a gene, but several genes could be transferred as well — from one (or more) species into the genome of another is carried out. This type of transfer is called horizontal or lateral transfer of genetic material and cannot take place between the species involved in transgenesis as they are not capable of sexual reproduction with each other — *that is.* vertical transfer. So, in essence, transgenic technology introduces novel genes into an organism in order to enhance it with new characteristics. On the other hand, most of the gene editing tools act on the genetic material of a single organism (and species) and their genetic and phenotypic effects are the same as in the case of naturally, spontaneous occurring mutations. It should be noted that the transfer of novel genes — just like in the case of transgenesis — is also possible.

Authors do not always make the same distinction between GE, transgenesis, and genome editing. Often, GE and transgenesis were used interchangeably, especially before genome editing became widespread. Today, such an approach can be somewhat confusing — "advancements in genetic engineering and genome editing techniques draw more attention from conventional plant breeding methods" [78] — and there are many other examples that may hinder even more the understanding of the differences between the three concepts mentioned earlier:

- "The process of genetic engineering or gene editing in plants starts with isolation of the desired gene from a living source, which is then incorporated within a suitable vector to make a recombinant DNA molecule, and finally this recombinant DNA molecule is inserted into the host's (plant) genome — thus integrating a new function within the GM plant. One of the main components of gene editing tools used for production of GM crops that have the most significant impact upon the overall process of gene editing is selection of a suitable enzyme." [79].

- "Gene editing can be defined as a process involving advanced techniques in molecular biology for site-specific, efficient, and precise modifications within a genome. The resultant plants can be precisely termed as genetically modified (GM) plants that occur through the transfer of a transgene (gene) of known function." [79].

In the following subchapters, general aspects regarding transgenesis and genome editing will be presented briefly.

4.2.1 Transgenic breeding

During the past four decades, the asexual transfer of genes employing specific GE methods has added a new dimension to the genetic modification and improvement of plants [57]. It should be noted that *genetic modification* is often used to refer specifically to genetic engineering and transgenesis [14, 80]. However, the term has traditionally been used to describe any heritable (genetic) improvements in plants (or animals) irrespective of the methodology employed by the breeders [14, 80]. Modifications — insertions, deletions, or substitutions — can range from small-scale alterations, such as a single nucleotide affecting a single gene to major changes in the genetic makeup, affecting numerous genes.

The products of GE — called transgenic plants or crops and commonly referred to as GM or biotech — became the most rapidly spreading agricultural technology in history [81, 82]. They contain at least one (foreign or exogenous) gene that has been artificially inserted into their genome to determine a desired characteristic [49, 77]. The inserted gene is known as a transgene [83] and originates from different sexually incompatible species or can even be completely artificially synthesized.

Consequently, transgenic technology can overcome the reproductive barriers of transferring genetic material so that breeding resources are extended to unrelated species, creating additional genetic variation [49, 77, 84] — characteristics not available in nature in the plants to be modified are introduced from a variety of other organisms [3, 57]. In this way, transgenesis is fundamentally different from traditional, mutation-based, or molecular marker-based breeding [57]. Such an approach also produces plants with desired characteristics faster than classical breeding [3], enabling the insertion of the foreign DNA directly into elite cultivars (genotypes) [49, 83]. The two most popular techniques for plant transformation are *Agrobacterium*-mediated gene transfer (plant transformation) and particle bombardment [75, 84].

Two particular types of transgenesis have been developed for transferring DNA that belongs to the same species or to other closely related and sexually compatible species: cisgenesis employs natural genetic sequences (i.e. genes with their regulatory elements) for genetic modification, while intragenesis refers to the use of new combinations of coding sequences and regulatory elements [77, 85]. There are different goals for these types of transfers —*for example.* Overexpression of genes that are already present within the crop itself, avoiding linkage drag that occurs when gene transfer is obtained by crossing — but a very important aspect is that the gene pool exploited by these approaches is identical to the gene pool available for traditional breeding. In this way, objections to transgenesis may be overcome more easily [77].

Gene silencing is another important tool used in plant transgenesis [86], encompassing a series of mechanisms capable of suppressing or inhibiting gene expression [83, 86].

4.2.2 Genome editing

Several new (plant) breeding techniques (NPBTs or NBTs) — also termed novel genomic techniques, new genetic modification techniques, etc. — have been developed over the past few decades [32, 33, 36, 87]. NBTs is an umbrella term, encompassing different biotechnological approaches employed in research and breeding that are capable modifying an organism's genetic makeup and that have emerged or have been created since 2001 [32, 33, 36]. Of these, genome editing or gene editing (GEd), is a particularly useful strategy for the genetic improvement of crops, allowing much faster and more precise results than other breeding techniques [32, 33, 77]. Therefore, GEd has evolved rapidly in recent years, and it has received increasingly more attention [77, 88, 89], both from researchers and the general public, not only in plant breeding but also in many other research areas as well.

There are many different molecular (genome) editors available, such as site-directed nucleases (SDNs), which include meganucleases (MNs), zinc-finger nucleases (ZFNs), transcription activator-like effector nucleases (TALENs) and CRISPR/Cas or CRISPR-Cas systems — CRISPR is an acronym for clustered regularly interspaced short palindromic repeat, while Cas stands for CRISPR-associated protein, prime editing (PE), base editing (BE), oligonucleotide-directed mutagenesis (ODM), transposases, recombinases, chemical (chemistry-based) DNA cutters, and peptide nucleic acids (PNAs) [90–92]. Although some editing systems have been introduced since the 1990s, with the first one even earlier, it was the CRISPR/Cas-based platform that really "revolutionized this revolutionary field." Introduced only in 2013, the CRISPR/Cas technology became, by far, the most popular tool for editing the genetic blueprint of an organism due to its simplicity and versatility — CRISPR/Cas can be easily adapted and programmed for many different uses — and continues to drive major breakthroughs in life sciences [90, 93]. The four main classes of CRISPR/Cas-derived genome editors are nucleases (*i.e.* SDNs), base editors (*i.e.* BE), prime editors (*i.e.* PE), and transposases/recombinases [90].

In essence, GEd systems generate targeted DNA mutations (at predefined locations in the genome) [49, 94], ranging from one or a few nucleotides, just like naturally occurring mutations, to inserting or removing one or more entirely functional genes [9, 36, 37].

Applications of SDNs-based GEd — mainly CRISPR/Cas — are generally grouped into different types — SDN-1, SDN-2, and SDN-3 — depending on the presence of exogenous DNA, the cellular response mechanism, and the resulting change in the genetic makeup of the targeted organism [89, 93, 95, 96]. SDN-1 and SDN-2 are somewhat similar, producing plants that contain no exogenous DNA in their genome. The desired traits result from changes, such as nucleotide substitutions and small deletions and insertions, made exclusively on endogenous DNA and are indistinguishable from natural genetic variation or what can be obtained by mutation breeding [9, 95]. The European Network of GMO Laboratories concluded that without prior knowledge, it is technically impossible to detect the small DNA changes introduced by Ged, and thus to distinguish GEd plants from plants selected for certain naturally occurring mutations or plants that are obtained through mutation breeding [9, 33]. SDN-3, on the other hand, results in the insertion of exogenous DNA into the target genome at a predefined locus, and such organisms are considered to be GMOs [9, 95]. PE and BE constitute separate categories than any SDN, but the genetic changes they are producing are similar to SDN-1 and SDN-2 [9].

Breeding has always relied heavily on genetic diversity and modern breeders have continuously looked for ways to expand it [9]. So, over time, breeding efforts were augmented by introducing various means — *that is.* artificial mutagenesis and trangenesis — for creating new genetic variants in addition to the spontaneous mutations found in nature [9]. One of the drawbacks of artificially induced mutations is that it generates many (probably thousands) unknown and uncontrolled mutations in a genome, even deleterious ones, so isolating a desired new trait could still be time-consuming and, in some cases, virtually impossible [9, 77]. In this context, a distinction must be made between undirected methods — *that is.* artificial mutation methods causing random genetic changes — and the more precise site-directed methods [97] — *that is.* GEd, also called targeted genome engineering [94]. So, unlike artificial mutations, the changes produced by GEd are not random, being targeted at a specific predetermined locus, which gives this technology a high level of precision while generating new variability [9]. Therefore, GEd increases the efficiency of introducing single and multiple traits and removing undesirable ones without affecting genetically linked genes [37].

In many countries, the development, commercialization, and use of GM crops are severely limited due to the many regulatory, social, and ethical issues and concerns related to environmental safety and consumer health [9, 77]. As pointed out before, most GEd technologies work without introducing exogenous DNA fragments in the targeted genome and their effects on the DNA and phenotype are the same as those of conventional mutations. It can thus be concluded that "the process is genetic engineering, but the product is not" [97], which should contribute to their acceptance. Certain authors go as far as calling GEd technology and organisms transgene-free [76, 98]. In fact, one of the most intriguing aspects related to GEd is its legal status, especially in relation to transgenesis — whether or not it falls in the same category as GMOs. Two major rulings applicable GEd were issued in 2018:

1. The US did not regulate "plants that could otherwise have been developed through traditional breeding techniques" because they are considered "indistinguishable from those developed through traditional breeding methods;" so, in the US, gene editing is not part of the same regulatory oversite as GMOs; a key point in this regard is the fact that it is nearly impossible to detect whether an organism's DNA has been edited [9, 36, 93, 95, 99]. As a result, several countries worldwide have fully or partially exempted from national biosafety regulations specific types of GEd organisms [95].

2. The ruling of the European Court of Justice (Case C-528/16) was interpreted by the European authorities to mean that organisms developed through so-called NBT, including GEd crops are not excluded from the scope of the legislation on GMOs — Directive 2001/18/EC; this opinion is based on the fact that GEd techniques alter the genome in such a way that would not occur naturally or by mating, and they do not have a long safety record [9, 36, 37, 93, 95, 99].

The European regulatory approach regarding GEd crops is considered to be completely out of line with the regulations existing in other countries [9] and may constitute an important barrier for GEd-based research and the varieties obtained by GEd [9, 36]. There is a growing consensus that risk assessment should differentiate between GEd crops that have DNA changes, which can also occur spontaneously in nature or as a result of conventional breeding, and Ged crops having genome changes, which cannot occur in nature or as a result of conventional breeding methods — *that is.* the insertion of a foreign gene to a predefined location in the genome (SDN-3).

Despite the tremendous potential and the promising results obtained so far, there are still enough technical hurdles that need to be overcome so that the utility of GEd can be exploited as best as possible and with as few negative consequences as possible [97]. There are continuous efforts for streamlining the delivery of editing system components into cells and for preventing off-target effects — improving the specificity or efficiency of producing only the desired edits [37, 95]. Nevertheless, it should be taken into consideration that, in plants, the off-target modifications are a relative discussion in the context of mutation breeding methods, which create many more random changes to the genome [9].

GEd arguably represents the most dynamic and rapidly evolving sector of GE and biotechnology, with new applications being published almost daily [9]. Researchers have adopted GEd technology at an unprecedented speed because of its high precision, time and cost efficiency, simplicity, and versatility that accelerated the plant breeding process — genetic variations determining a certain favorable trait are introduced in one or two generations of plants [37, 49, 77]. There is a broad consensus that GEd crops will make a critical contribution to agriculture — and to other areas as well — in the coming years [9]. But the way GEd crops are regulated internationally — whether they fall under the scope of GMO legislation or not — will have a significant impact on the development of GEd technologies and their potential to benefit mankind [77].

5. Concluding remarks

As long as the human population continues to grow, there will also be a high demand for agricultural products. Increased production can be achieved by expanding the cultivated land area, using appropriate agronomic practices (*e.g.* fertilizers, irrigation, and crop rotation) and cultivating superior plant varieties. However, farmlands are sometimes converted to other uses because an increasing population comes with higher needs for residential, commercial, industrial, and recreational land uses. There are also more and more limitations on available resources and protecting the environment should be taken very seriously in the coming years. In this context, the challenge is to improve agricultural yields while decreasing the use of resources. The solution to this challenge rests with the genotypes being cultivated. Developing varieties superior to the already existing ones is achieved by plant breeding, which, in its modern form, is a very systematic and highly technological approach.

Humans have carried out plant breeding since they first started farming, but its scientific basis was firmly established only at the beginning of the twentieth century when Mendel's work on heredity and variability was rediscovered. Since then, science and technology have made plant breeding more and more efficient, and spectacular advances have been made by breeders after the implementation of new molecular and biotechnological knowledge over the past few decades.

Plant breeding simultaneously enhances and exploits biological diversity — *that is.* genetic variation. Therefore, many achievements in plant breeding were based on phenotypic selection, which is still widely used. However, traditional breeding is becoming more sophisticated with the addition of modern strategies. The initial integration of molecular markers in plant breeding — marker-assisted selection — allowed important progress to be made, and now, due to the availability and employment of new sequencing technologies, genomic-based approaches are likely to dramatically change the selection process.

Traditional breeding primarily exploits natural genetic variation, and mutation breeding and genome editing were designed to extend this type of variation, but not beyond species limitations. Further expansion of variability beyond the natural boundaries of sexual reproduction was enabled by other advances in molecular biology and biotechnology — transgenesis allows the transfer of genes between sexually incompatible species. In this way, there is essentially one universal gene pool from which breeders may obtain variability for crop improvement.

The implementation of the new approaches presented in this chapter has already made invaluable contributions to overcoming the aforementioned agricultural threats and challenges. Other possibilities of augmenting breeding methodologies that have not been discussed here are also available: metabolomics-assisted breeding, high-throughput or automated phenotyping, RNA and epigenetic editing (*i.e.* modification), etc.

This chapter provided an introduction to plant breeding by presenting the main types of genetic improvement that were devised to meet the needs of an ever-growing human civilization. There is a large variety of tools available to breeders, both simple and complex, with incredible advantages but also drawbacks. The information is, thus, a vital resource for students interested in this field of agricultural sciences.

Author details

Cristian-Radu Sisea*
Faculty of Horticulture and Business in Rural Development, University of Agricultural Sciences and Veterinary Medicine Cluj-Napoca, Cluj-Napoca, Romania

*Address all correspondence to: cristian.sisea@usamvcluj.ro

References

[1] Ha M, Schleiger R. Selective Breeding and Genetic Engineering [Internet]. Davis, CA, USA: LibreTexts, Inc.; 2023. Available from: https://bio.libretexts.org/Bookshelves/Ecology/Environmental_Science_(Ha_and_Schleiger)/04%3A_Humans_and_the_Environment/4.03%3A_Agriculture/4.3.03%3A_Selective_Breeding_and_Genetic_Engineering [Accessed: Sep. 23, 2023]

[2] Gepts P. A comparison between crop domestication, classical plant breeding, and genetic engineering. Crop Science. 2002;**42**(6):1780-1790. DOI: 10.2135/cropsci2002.1780

[3] Priyadarshan PM. Plant Breeding: Classical to Modern. Singapore: Springer Nature Singapore Pte Ltd; 2019. 570 p. DOI: 10.1007/978-981-13-7095-3

[4] Acquaah G. Principles of Plant Genetics and Breeding. 2nd ed. Chichester, West Sussex, UK: John Wiley & Sons, Ltd; 2012. 740 p. DOI: 10.1002/9781118313718

[5] Acquaah G. Conventional plant breeding principles and techniques. In: Al-Khayri JM, Jain SM, Johnson DV, editors. Advances in Plant Breeding Strategies: Breeding, Biotechnology and Molecular Tools. Vol. 1. Switzerland: Springer International Publishing; 2015. pp. 115-158. DOI: 10.1007/978-3-319-22521-0

[6] Orton TJ. Horticultural Plant Breeding. London, United Kingdom: Academic Press; 2020. 397 p. DOI: 10.1016/C2017-0-03393-1

[7] Fehr WR. Principles of Cultivar Development. In: Theory and Technique. Vol. 1. New York: Macmillan Publishing Company; 1987. 536 p

[8] Bharadwaj DN. Sustainable agriculture and food security: 2050 (future plant breeding). In: Bharadwaj DN, editor. Advanced Molecular Plant Breeding: Meeting the Challenge of Food Security. New-York: Apple Academic Press; 2018. pp. 3-30. DOI: 10.1201/b22473

[9] Dima O, Bocken H, Custers R, Inze D, Puigdomènech P. Genome editing for crop improvement. In: Symposium Summary. Berlin: ALLEA – All European Academies; 2020. 64 p. DOI: 10.26356/gen-editing-crop

[10] Lobato-Gómez M, Hewitt S, Capell T, Christou P, Dhingra A, Girón-Calva PS. Transgenic and genome-edited fruits: Background, constraints, benefits, and commercial opportunities. Horticulture Research. 2021;**8**:166. DOI: 10.1038/s41438-021-00601-3

[11] Varshney RK, Bohra A, Yu J, Graner A, Zhang Q, Sorrells ME. Designing future crops: Genomics-assisted breeding comes of age. Trends in Plant Science. 2021;**26**(6):631-649. DOI: 10.1016/j.tplants.2021.03.010

[12] Sleper DA, Poehlman JM. Breeding Field Crops. 5th ed. Oxford: Blackwell Publishing; 2006. 424 p. DOI: 10.1007/978-94-015-7271-2

[13] Voss-Fels KP, Stahl A, Hickey LT. Q&A: Modern crop breeding for future food security. BMC Biology. 2019;**17**. DOI: 10.1186/s12915-019-0638-4

[14] U.S. Department of Agriculture. Agricultural Biotechnology Glossary [Internet]. Available from: https://www.usda.gov/topics/biotechnology/

biotechnology-glossary [Accessed: Sep. 07, 2023]

[15] Moose SP, Mumm RH. Molecular plant breeding as the foundation for 21st century crop improvement. Plant Physiology. 2008;**147**(3):969-977. DOI: 10.1104/pp.108.118232

[16] Koh HJ, Kwon SY, Thomson M, editors. Current Technologies in Plant Molecular Breeding – A Guide Book of Plant Molecular Breeding for Researchers. New York. London: Springer Science+Business Media Dordrecht; 2015. 360 p. DOI: 10.1007/978-94-017-9996-6

[17] Khan S, Pandotra P, Gupta AP, Salgotra RK, Manzoor MM, Lone SA, et al. Plant molecular breeding: Way forward through next-generation sequencing. In: Zargar SM, Rai V, editors. Plant Omics and Crop Breeding. Waretown, NJ, USA: Apple Academic Press Inc.; 2017. pp. 201-234. DOI: 10.1201/9781315365930

[18] Mehta DR, Nandha AK. Terminator technology (GURT technology). In: Bharadwaj DN, editor. Advanced Molecular Plant Breeding: Meeting the Challenge of Food Security. New-York: Apple Academic Press; 2018. pp. 505-534. DOI: 10.1201/b22473

[19] Anand A, Subramanian M, Kar D. Breeding techniques to dispense higher genetic gains. Frontiers in Plant Science. 2023;**13**:1076094. DOI: 10.3389/fpls.2022.1076094

[20] Chahal GS, Gosal SS. Principles and procedures of plant breeding. In: Biotechnological and Conventional Approaches. Harrow: Alpha Science International; 2002. 604 p

[21] International Service for the Acquisition of Agri-biotech Applications. Agricultural biotechnology – A lot more than just GM crops [Internet]. 2014. Available from: https://www.isaaa.org/resources/publications/agricultural_biotechnology/download/agricultural_biotechnology.pdf [Accessed: Sep. 11, 2023]

[22] Rai GK, Kumar RR, Bagati S, editors. Abiotic Stress Tolerance Mechanisms in Plants. London: CRC Press; 2021. 370 p. DOI: 10.1201/9781003163831

[23] van de Wiel C, Schaart J, Niks R, Visser R. Traditional Plant Breeding Methods. Wageningen UR Plant Breeding: Wageningen; 2010. 66 p

[24] Budhlakoti N, Kushwaha AK, Rai A, Chaturvedi KK, Kumar A, Pradhan AK, et al. Genomic selection: A tool for accelerating the efficiency of molecular breeding for development of climate-resilient crops. Frontiers in Genetics. 2022;**13**:832153. DOI: 10.3389/fgene.2022.832153

[25] Breseghello F, Coelho AS. Traditional and modern plant breeding methods with examples in rice (*Oryza sativa* L.). Journal of Agricultural and Food Chemistry. 2013;**61**(35):8277-8286. DOI: 10.1021/jf305531j

[26] International Service for the Acquisition of Agri-biotech Applications. Pocket K No. 13: Conventional plant breeding [Internet]. 2006. Available from: https://www.isaaa.org/resources/publications/pocketk/13/default.asp [Accessed: Sep. 19, 2023]

[27] Sarsu F, Penna S, Kunter B, Ibrahim R. Mutation breeding for vegetatively propagated crops. In: Spencer-Lopes MM, Forster BP, Jankuloski L, editors. Manual on Mutation Breeding. 3rd ed. Rome: Food and Agriculture Organization of the United Nations; 2018. pp. 157-176

[28] Datta SK. Induced Mutation Breeding. Singapore: Springer Nature Singapore Pte Ltd.; 2023. 179 p. DOI: 10.1007/978-981-19-9489-0

[29] Penna S, Jain SM. Mutation Breeding for Sustainable Food Production and Climate Resilience. Singapore: Springer Nature Singapore Pte Ltd.; 2023. 815 p. DOI: 10.1007/978-981-16-9720-3

[30] Ahmar S, Gill RA, Jung KH, Faheem A, Qasim MU, Mubeen M, et al. Conventional and molecular techniques from simple breeding to speed breeding in crop plants: Recent advances and future outlook. International Journal of Molecular Sciences. 2020;**21**(7):2590. DOI: 10.3390/ijms21072590

[31] Spencer-Lopes MM, Forster BP, Jankuloski L. Manual on Mutation Breeding. 3rd ed. Rome: Food and Agriculture Organization of the United Nations; 2018. 301 p

[32] Laaninen T. New plant-breeding techniques. Applicability of EU GMO rules [Internet]. 2019. Available from: https://www.europarl.europa.eu/RegData/etudes/BRIE/2019/642235/EPRS_BRI(2019)642235_EN.pdf [Accessed: Sep. 19, 2023]

[33] Laaninen T. New plant-breeding techniques. Applicability of EU GMO rules [Internet]. 2020. Available from: https://www.europarl.europa.eu/RegData/etudes/BRIE/2020/659343/EPRS_BRI(2020)659343_EN.pdf [Accessed: Sep. 19, 2023]

[34] Okole B, Memela C, Rademan S, Kunert KJ, Brunette M. Non-conventional breeding approaches for banana and plantain improvement against fungal diseases at AECI. Acta Horticulturae. 2000;**540**:207-214. DOI: 10.17660/ActaHortic.2000.540.23

[35] Chen YF, Dai XM, Gong Q, Huang X, Xiao W, Zhao JT, et al. Non-conventional breeding of banana (*Musa* spp.). Acta Horticulturae. 2011;**897**:39-46. DOI: 10.17660/actahortic.2011.897.2

[36] Van der Meer P, Angenon G, Bergmans H, Buhk HJ, Callebaut S, Chamon M, et al. The status under EU law of organisms developed through novel genomic techniques. European Journal of Risk Regulation. 2020;**14**(1):93-112

[37] The Parliamentary Office of Science and Technology. Genome-Edited Food Crops [Internet]. Westminster, London: The Parliamentary Office of Science and Technology; 2022. Available from: https://researchbriefings.files.parliament.uk/documents/POST-PN-0663/POST-PN-0663.pdf [Accessed: Sep. 19, 2023]

[38] Mallikarjuna MG, Veeraya P, Tomar R, Jha S, Nayaka SC, Lohithaswa HC, et al. Next-generation breeding approaches for stress resilience in cereals: Current status and future prospects. In: Mallikarjuna MG, Nayaka SC, Kaul T, editors. Next-Generation Plant Breeding Approaches for Stress Resilience in Cereal Crops. Singapore: Springer Nature Singapore Pte Ltd.; 2022. pp. 1-44. DOI: 10.1007/978-981-19-1445-4

[39] Babu HP, Kumar M, Gaikwad KB, Kumar R, Kumar N, Palaparthi D, et al. Rapid generation advancement and fast-track breeding approaches in wheat improvement. In: Mallikarjuna MG, Nayaka SC, Kaul T, editors. Next-Generation Plant Breeding Approaches for Stress Resilience in Cereal Crops. Singapore: Springer Nature Singapore Pte Ltd.; 2022. pp. 241-262. DOI: 10.1007/978-981-19-1445-4

[40] Chimmili SR, Kanneboina S, Hanjagi PS, Basavaraj PS, Sakhare AS,

Senguttuvel P, et al. Integrating advanced molecular, genomic, and speed breeding methods for genetic improvement of stress tolerance in rice. In: Mallikarjuna MG, Nayaka SC, Kaul T, editors. Next-Generation Plant Breeding Approaches for Stress Resilience in Cereal Crops. Singapore: Springer Nature Singapore Pte Ltd.; 2022. pp. 263-284. DOI: 10.1007/978-981-19-1445-4

[41] Singh H, Janeja HS. Speed breeding a ray of hope for the future generation in terms of food security: A review. Plant Archives. 2021;**21**(1):155-158. DOI: 10.51470/plantarchives.2021.v21.s1.028

[42] Wanga MA, Shimelis H, Mashilo J, Laing MD. Opportunities and challenges of speed breeding: A review. Plant Breeding. 2021;**140**(2):185-194. DOI: 10.1111/pbr.12909

[43] Malik B, Pirzadah TB, Qureshi I, Tahir I, Murtaza I, Rehman RU. Phenomics science: An integrated inter-disciplinary approach for crop improvement. In: Zargar SM, Rai V, editors. Plant OMICS and Crop Breeding. Oakville: Apple Academic Press; 2017. pp. 201-234. DOI: 10.1201/9781315365930

[44] Tripodi P. Crop breeding. In: Methods in Molecular Biology. New York, NY, USA: Springer Science+Business Media, LLC; 2018. 282 p. DOI: 10.1007/978-1-0716-1201-9

[45] Boopathi NM, Sathish S, Kavitha P, Dachinamoorthy P, Ravikesavan R. Molecular breeding for genetic improvement of cotton (*Gossypium* spp.). In: Al-Khayri JM, Jain SM, Johnson DV, editors. Advances in Plant Breeding Strategies: Breeding, Biotechnology and Molecular Tools. Vol. 1. Switzerland: Springer International Publishing; 2015. DOI: 10.1007/978-3-319-22521-0

[46] Mahajan R, Nazir M, Sayeed N, Rai V, Mushtaq R, Masoodi KZ, et al. Unraveling the abiotic stress tolerance in common bean through omics. In: Zargar SM, Rai V, editors. Plant Omics and Crop Breeding. Oakville: Apple Academic Press; 2017. pp. 313-368. DOI: 10.1201/9781315365930 311-365

[47] Jiang GL. Molecular markers and marker-assisted breeding in plants. In: Andersen SB, editor. Plant Breeding from Laboratories to Fields. London, United Kingdom: IntechOpen; 2013. pp. 45-83. DOI: 10.5772/52583

[48] Jiang GL. Molecular markers and marker-assisted breeding in plants. In: Al-Khayri JM, Jain SM, Johnson DV, editors. Advances in Plant Breeding Strategies: Breeding, Biotechnology and Molecular Tools. Vol. 1. Switzerland: Springer International Publishing; 2015. pp. 431-472. DOI: 10.1007/978-3-319-22521-0

[49] Gaur RK, Verma RK, Khurana SMP. Genetic Engineering of Horticultural Crops: Present and Future. In: Rout GR, Peter KV, editors. London: Academic Press; 2018. 444 p

[50] Rai R, Singh AK, Zargar SM, Singh DB. A recap on quantitative trait loci associated with disease resistance in food legumes. In: Zargar SM, Rai V, editors. Plant Omics and Crop Breeding. Oakville, ON, Canada: Apple Academic Press Inc.; 2017. 495 p. DOI: 10.1201/9781315365930

[51] Kaur L, Meena MR, Lenka SK, Appunu C, Kumar R, Kulshreshtha N. Molecular approaches for improving abiotic stress tolerance in sugarcane. In: Shanker AK, Shanker C, Anand A, Maheswari M, editors. Climate Change and Crop Stress. Molecules to Ecosistems. London, United Kingdom: Academic

Press; 2021. pp. 465-492. DOI: 10.1016/C2017-0-03584-X

[52] Nataraja KN, Madhura BG, Parvathi MS. Omics: Modern tools for precise understanding of drought adaptation in plants. In: Zargar SM, Rai V, editors. Plant Omics and Crop Breeding. Oakville, ON, Canada: Apple Academic Press Inc.; 2017. pp. 263-294. DOI: 10.1201/9781315365930

[53] Jaradat AA. Breeding oilseed crops for climate change. In: Jaradat AA, editor. Breeding Oilseed Crops for Sustainable Production. London, United Kingdom: Academic Press; 2016. pp. 421-472. DOI: 10.1016/B978-0-12-801309-0.00018-5

[54] Lodhi SS, Maryam S, Rafique K, Shafique A, Yousaf ZA, Talha AM, et al. Overview of the prospective strategies for conservation of genomic diversity in wheat landraces. In: Climate Change and Food Security with Emphasis on Wheat. London, United Kingdom: Academic Press; 2020. pp. 293-309. DOI: 10.1016/B978-0-12-819527-7.0021-2

[55] Al-Khayri JM, Jain SM, Johnson DV. Advances in Plant Breeding Strategies: Breeding, Biotechnology and Molecular Tools. Vol. 1. Switzerland: Springer International Publishing; 2015. 656 p. DOI: 10.1007/978-3-319-22521-0

[56] Agnihotri A, Kumar M, Kilam D, Aneja JK. Genomic and transcriptomic approaches for quality improvement in oilseed brassicas. In: Plant OMICS and Crop Breeding. Oakville, ON, Canada: Apple Academic Press Inc.; 2017. pp. 31-48. DOI: 10.1201/9781315365930

[57] White TL, Adams WT, Neale DB. Forest Genetics. Cambridge: CABI Publishing; 2007. 702 p. DOI: 10.1079/9781845932855.0000

[58] Koh HJ, Kwon SY, Thomson M, editors. Current Technologies in Plant Molecular Breeding. A Guide Book of Plant Molecular Breeding for Researchers. New York. London: Springer Science+Business Media Dordrecht; 2015. p. 360. DOI: 10.1007/978-94-017-9996-6

[59] Bhat JA, Ali S, Salgotra RK, Mir ZA, Dutta S, Jadon V, et al. Genomic selection in the era of next generation sequencing for complex traits in plant breeding. Frontiers in Genetics. 2016;7:221. DOI: 10.3389/fgene.2016.00221

[60] Leng PF, Lübberstedt T, Xu ML. Genomics-assisted breeding–a revolutionary strategy for crop improvement. Journal of Integrative Agriculture. 2017;**16**(12):2674-2685. DOI: 10.1016/S2095-3119(17)61813-6

[61] Ashraf M, Akram NA, Foolad MR. Marker-assisted selection in plant breeding for salinity tolerance. In: Walker J, editor. Plant Salt Tolerance: Methods and Protocols. Totowa, NJ: Humana Press; 2012. pp. 305-333

[62] Kang M, Ahn H, Rothe E, Baldwin IT, Kim SG. A robust genome-editing method for wild plant species *Nicotiana attenuata*. Plant Biotechnology Reports. 2020;**14**:585-598. DOI: 10.1007/s11816-020-00634-5

[63] Hasan N, Choudhary S, Naaz N, Sharma N, Laskar RA. Recent advancements in molecular marker-assisted selection and applications in plant breeding programmes. Journal of Genetic Engineering and Biotechnology. 2021;**19**(1):1-26. DOI: 10.1186/s43141-021-00231-1

[64] Dekkers JC, Hospital F. The use of molecular genetics in the improvement of agricultural populations. Nature Reviews Genetics. 2002;**3**(1):22-32. DOI: 10.1038/nrg701

[65] Beuzen ND, Stear MJ, Chang KC. Molecular markers and their use in animal breeding. The Veterinary Journal. 2000;**160**(1):42-52. DOI: 10.1053/tvjl.2000.0468

[66] Yadav AK, Tomar SS, Jha AK, Singh J. Importance of molecular markers in livestock improvement: A review. International Journal of Agriculture Innovations and Research. 2017;**5**(4):614-622

[67] Singh U, Deb R, Alyethodi RR, Alex R, Kumar S, Chakraborty S, et al. Molecular markers and their applications in cattle genetic research: A review. Biomarkers and Genomic Medicine. 2014;**6**(2):49-58. DOI: 10.1016/j.bgm.2014.03.001

[68] Amiteye S. Basic concepts and methodologies of DNA marker systems in plant molecular breeding. Heliyon. 2021;**7**(10). DOI: 10.1016/j.heliyon.2021.e08093

[69] Chaudhary HK, Badiyal A, Hussain W, Jamwal NS, Kumar N, Sharma P, et al. Innovative role of DH breeding in genomics assisted-crop improvement: Focus on drought tolerance in wheat. In: Rajpal V, Sehgal D, Kumar A, Raina S, editors. Genomics Assisted Breeding of Crops for Abiotic Stress Tolerance, Vol. II., Sustainable Development and Biodiversity. Vol. 21. Cham, Switzerland: Springer Nature Switzerland AG; 2019. pp. 91-103. DOI: 10.1007/978-3-319-99573-1_6

[70] Kumar S, Muthusamy SK, Mishra CN, Gupta V, Venkatesh K. Importance of genomic selection in crop improvement and future prospects. In: Bharadwaj DN, editor. Advanced Molecular Plant Breeding: Meeting the Challenge of Food Security. New-York: Apple Academic Press; 2018. pp. 505-534. DOI: 10.1201/b22473Oakville

[71] Visioni A, Al-Abdallat A, Elenien JA, Verma RPS, Gyawali S, Baum M. Genomics and molecular breeding for improving tolerance to abiotic stress in barley (*Hordeum vulgare* L.). In: Rajpal V, Sehgal D, Kumar A, Raina S, editors. Genomics Assisted Breeding of Crops for Abiotic Stress Tolerance, Vol. II, Sustainable Development and Biodiversity. Vol. 21. Cham, Switzerland: Springer Nature Switzerland AG; 2019. pp. 49-68. DOI: 10.1007/978-3-319-99573-1_6

[72] Skøt L, Kelly R, Humphreys MW. Genomics assisted approaches for improving abiotic stress tolerance in forage grasses. In: Rajpal V, Sehgal D, Kumar A, Raina S, editors. Genomics Assisted Breeding of Crops for Abiotic Stress Tolerance, Vol. II., Sustainable Development and Biodiversity. Vol. 21. Cham, Switzerland: Springer Nature Switzerland AG; 2019. pp. 91-103. DOI: 10.1007/978-3-319-99573-1_6

[73] Chaudhary J, Alisha A, Bhatt V, Chandanshive S, Kumar N, Mir Z, et al. Mutation breeding in tomato: Advances, applicability and challenges. Plants. 2019;**8**(5):128. DOI: 10.3390/plants8050128

[74] Okada T, Whitford R. Hybrid wheat and abiotic stress. In: Rajpal V, Sehgal D, Kumar A, Raina SN, editors. Genomics Assisted Breeding of Crops for Abiotic Stress Tolerance. Vol. II. Cham, Switzerland: Springer Nature Switzerland AG; 2019. pp. 211-224. DOI: 10.1007/978-3-319-99573-1_6

[75] Agarwal S, Grover A, Khurana SMP. Plant molecular biology: Tools to develop transgenics. In: Khan MS, Khan AI, Barh D, editors. Applied Molecular Biotechnology. The Next Generation of Genetic Engineering. Boca Raton, FL, USA: CRC Press; 2016. pp. 33-60

[76] Lawrenson T, Atkinson N, Forner M, Harwood W. Highly efficient gene knockout in medicago truncatula genotype R108 using CRISPR-Cas9 system and an optimized agrobacterium transformation method. In: Yang B, Harwood W, Que Q, editors. Plant Genome Engineering: Methods and Protocols. 2023. pp. 221-252. DOI: 10.1007/978-1-0716-3131-7_15

[77] Marone D, Mastrangelo AM, Borrelli GM. From transgenesis to genome editing in crop improvement: Applications, marketing, and legal issues. International Journal of Molecular Sciences. 2023;**24**(8):7122. DOI: 10.3390/ijms24087122

[78] Shackira AM, Sarath NG, Veena M, Johnson R, Jeyaraj S, Aswathy Raj KP, et al. Resistance identification and implementation. In: Shah T, Nie L, Teixeira Filho MCM, Amir R, editors. Cereal Crops: Genetic Resources and Breeding Techniques. Boca Raton, FL, USA: CRC Press; 2023. pp. 141-156. DOI: 10.1201/9781003250845

[79] Ahad A, Jan US, Rafique K, Zafar S, Ahmad MA, Abbas F, et al. Climate change and cereal modeling. Impacts and adaptability. In: Shah T, Nie L, Teixeira Filho MC, Amir R, editors. Cereal Crops: Genetic Resources and Breeding Techniques. Boca Raton, FL, USA: CRC Press; 2023. pp. 239-272. DOI: 10.1201/9781003250845

[80] U.S. Food and Drug Administration. Voluntary Labeling Indicating Whether Foods Have or Have Not Been Derived from Genetically Engineered Plants: Guidance for Industry [Internet]. 2019. Available from: https://www.fda.gov/media/120958/download?attachment [Accessed: Sep. 19, 2023]

[81] Raney T. Economic impact of transgenic crops in developing countries. Current Opinion in Biotechnology. 2006;**17**(2):174-178. DOI: 10.1016/j.copbio.2006.02.009

[82] James C. Global Status of Commercialized Biotech/GM Crops. Brief 44. ISAAA: Ithaca; 2012. 329 p

[83] Singh Y, Prajapati S. Status of horticultural crops: Identifying the need for transgenic traits. In: Rout GR, Peter KV, editors. Genetic Engineering of Horticultural Crops. London, United Kingdom: Academic Press; 2018. pp. 1-22

[84] Joung YH, Choi PS, SY K, Harn CH. Plant transformation methods and applications. In: Koh HJ, Kwon SY, Thomson M, editors. Current Technologies in Plant Molecular Breeding – A Guide Book of Plant Molecular Breeding for Researchers. New York. London: Springer Science+Business Media Dordrecht; 2015. pp. 296-344. DOI: 10.1007/978-94-017-9996-6

[85] Espinoza C, Schlechter R, Herrera D, Torres E, Serrano A, Medina C, et al. Cisgenesis and intragenesis: New tools for improving crops. Biological Research. 2013;**46**(4):323-331. DOI: 10.4067/S0716-97602013000400003

[86] Choudhary S, Jain D, Meena MR, Verma AK, Sharma R. Gene silencing in horticultural transgenic crops. In: Rout GR, Peter KV, editors. Genetic Engineering of Horticultural Crops. London, United Kingdom: Academic press; 2018. pp. 47-62

[87] Eckerstorfer MF, Engelhard M, Heissenberger A, Simon S, Teichmann H. Plants developed by new genetic modification techniques - Comparison of existing regulatory frameworks in the EU and non-EU countries. Frontiers in Bioengineering and Biotechnology. 2019;7:26. DOI: 10.3389/fbioe.2019.00026

[88] Cohen J. With its CRISPR Revolution, China Becomes a World Leader in Genome Editing. [Internet] Washington, DC, USA: American Association for the Advancement of Science; 2019. Available from: https://www.science.org/content/article/itscrispr-revolution-china-becomes-world-leader-genome-editing [Accessed: Sep. 19, 2023]

[89] Kuiken T, Kuzma J. Genome Editing in Latin America: Regional Regulatory Overview. Washington, DC, United States: Inter-American Development Bank; 2021. DOI: 10.18235/0003410

[90] Anzalone AV, Koblan LW, Liu DR. Genome editing with CRISPR–CAS nucleases, base editors, transposases and prime editors. Nature Biotechnology. 2020;**38**(7):824-844. DOI: 10.1038/s41587-020-0561-9

[91] Liu Z, Dong H, Cui Y, Cong L, Zhang D. Application of different types of CRISPR/Cas-based systems in bacteria. Microbial Cell Factories. 2020;**19**(1):1-4. DOI: 10.1186/s12934-020-01431-z

[92] Xu Y, Li Z. CRISPR-Cas systems: Overview, innovations and applications in human disease research and gene therapy. Computational and Structural Biotechnological Journal. 2020;**8**(18):2401-2415. DOI: 10.1016/j.csbj.2020.08.031

[93] Gocht A, Consmüller N, Thom F, Grethe H. Economic and environmental consequences of the ECJ genome editing judgment in agriculture. Agronomy. 2021;**11**(6):1212. DOI: 10.3390/agronomy11061212

[94] Kim H, Kim JS. A guide to genome engineering with programmable nucleases. Nature Reviews Genetics. 2014;**15**(5):321-334. DOI: 10.1038/nrg3686

[95] Rostoks N. Implications of the EFSA scientific opinion on site directed nucleases 1 and 2 for risk assessment of genome-edited plants in the EU. Agronomy. 2021;**11**(3):572. DOI: 10.3390/agronomy11030572

[96] Kawall K, Cotter J, Then C. Broadening the GMO risk assessment in the EU for genome editing technologies in agriculture. Environmental Sciences Europe. 2020;**32**(1):106. DOI: 10.1186/s12302-020-00361-2

[97] Wünschiers R. Genetic Engineering: Reading, Writing and Editing Genes. Wiesbaden, Germany: Springer Fachmedien Wiesbaden GmbH; 2021. 39 p

[98] Ma X, Li X, Li Z. Transgene-free genome editing in *Nicotiana benthamiana* with CRISPR/Cas9 delivered by a rhabdovirus vector. In: Yang B, Harwood W, Que Q, editors. Plant Genome Engineering: Methods and Protocols. 2023. pp. 173-185. DOI: 10.1007/978-1-0716-3131-7_11

[99] Schleissing S, Pfeilmeier S, Dürnberger C. An introduction: Between precaution and responsibility. In: Schleissing S, Pfeilmeier S, Dürnberger C, editors. Genome Editing in Agriculture: Between Precaution and Responsibility. Baden-Baden, Germany: Nomos; 2019. pp. 9-22. DOI: 10.5771/9783845296432-9

Chapter 2

Environmental Stress, Epigenetic Modifications, Adaptation, and Disease: A Fine Interplay

Maria Emileva Krasteva

Abstract

The epigenetic revolution has led to a paradigm shift in our understanding of gene regulation and function. Epigenetic modifications, including DNA methylation, post-translational histone modifications, and regulatory noncoding RNAs, display unique features, such as reversibility and transgenerational inheritance. A great variety of environmental and lifestyle factors can cause changes in the epigenome. Epigenetic alterations can contribute to the underlying mechanisms of human diseases including cancer, cardiovascular, neurological, psychiatric, autoimmune, metabolic and inherited. The chapter focuses on the fine interplay between environmental stress, the epigenetic adaptive responses, and how the inability to adapt may trigger disease outcomes. A model of the epigenetic disease is postulated, epigenetic disease adaptational model (EDAM), according to which the epigenetic disease develops as a failure to adapt to environmental stressors. This may occur in at least two possible scenarios: (1) when the epigenetic adaptational programs are not adequate to stress nature, duration, intensity and/or stage of action and (2) when the epigenetic adaptational programs are not adequate to the situation. In the second scenario, the stressful situation is wrongly considered the most feasible situation, and the stressful conditions are taken as "norm." The proposed model highlights important topics for future research in the field of epigenetics and disease.

Keywords: environmental stress, epigenetic modifications, gene expression, adaptive plasticity, epigenetic disease, epigenetic disease adaptational model (EDAM)

1. Introduction

The epigenetic revolution that has happened during the last decades has challenged our understanding of gene regulation and expression and has outlined the emergence of a new post-genomic era in biology. The long-term dogmatic views on heredity, exclusively relying on the genetic code inheritance, underwent significant scrutiny and questioning. The realization that the primary DNA sequence alone provides incomplete knowledge on the functioning of the genome has shifted the focus toward understanding the epigenetic processes, which modulate gene function by modifications in DNA or the associated proteins. This has been driven by advances in technology and methodologies such as DNA methylation profiling and chromatin immunoprecipitation that have allowed for precise mapping of epigenetic marks on a genome-wide scale. The definition of "epigenetics," originally introduced by Conrad Waddington in the early 1940s [1], as "the branch of biology, which studies the causal interactions between genes and their products, which bring the phenotype into being," has been notably evolved over time and now refers to "the study of changes in gene function that are heritable and that do not entail a change in DNA sequence" [2]. Epigenetic modifications ("epi" standing for "over" and "above") occur independent of the genetic sequence and provide an additional level of hereditary information denoted as "epigenetic code" [3]. The changes in the epigenome include three main classes: methylation in DNA, posttranslational histone modifications, and noncoding RNAs. Epigenetic changes, compared to genetic, display several unique characteristics including higher frequency, occurrence in specific genome regions, and potential reversibility. Evidence that comes from epigenetic research demonstrated that the genome is highly dynamic and responsive to environmental shifts. A great variety of environmental and lifestyle factors were shown to cause changes in the gene expression patterns mediated by epigenetics. With reference to this, epigenetic changes could be regarded as sensitive indicators of the interactions between the organism and the environment. Moreover, early embryogenesis is most vulnerable to epigenetic stress responses, at least some of which may increase the risk of malfunctioning and disease pathology in later life. Studies have shown transmission of environmentally induced epigenetic changes to the offspring in at least several species [4–6]. Though the evolutionarily significance of transgenerational epigenetics is still debatable, its significance for the organisms themselves and their near descendants seems quite feasible. In addition to their impact on various cellular processes, including shaping of cellular identity, development, and aging, epigenetic modifications were attributed a role in disease onset as well. Changes in the epigenome were related to many human disorders, such as cancer, cardiovascular diseases, neurological and psychiatric disorders, autoimmune diseases, metabolic diseases, and inherited disorders. This opened up possibilities for development of targeted interventions and therapeutic approaches, which can modulate gene expression patterns. Overall, the epigenetic revolution has led to a paradigm shift in our understanding of gene function by highlighting the dynamic nature and plasticity of how genes are regulated.

In this chapter, we provide an overview of the role of epigenetics in gene regulation, the impact of environmental and lifestyle factors on the epigenome, and the association between epigenetic modifications and various diseases. We propose the Epigenetic Disease Adaptational Model (EDAM) as a conceptual framework to elucidate how the inability to effectively adapt to environmental stressors may contribute to the development of epigenetic diseases. This model aims to provide insights into the complex interplay between the environment and the epigenome highlighting new possibilities for therapeutic approaches.

2. Types of epigenetic modifications

Three major mechanisms governing epigenetic regulation could be distinguished: methylation in DNA, posttranslational histone modifications (PTMs), and noncoding RNAs (ncRNAs). They modulate gene expression by causing changes in DNA-histones interactions responsible for the rearrangement of chromatin from a more open and transcriptionally accessible state (euchromatin) to a condensed chromatin structure that is transcriptionally less active (heterochromatin) and vice versa (**Figure 1**).

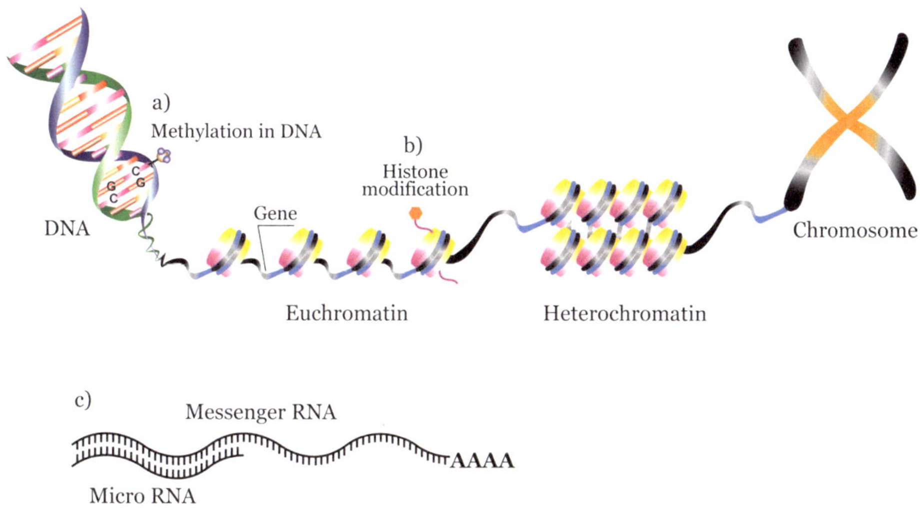

Figure 1.
Types of epigenetic modifications. (a) Methylation in DNA—Covalent attachment of a methyl group to the C5 position of cytosine residue in CpG dinucleotide sequences, (b) histone modifications—Posttranslational covalent addition of a chemical group (methylation, phosphorylation, acetylation, ubiquitylation, sumoylation), and (c) microRNAs (miRNAs)—Small noncoding RNAs which regulate post-transcriptional gene expression by binding to target mRNAs resulting in gene silencing. Epigenetic modifications regulate the dynamic transitions between transcriptionally active (euchromatin) or transcriptionally inactive (heterochromatin) states.

2.1 Methylation in DNA

Methylation in DNA is considered a relatively long term and stable epigenetic mark and can contribute to maintenance of cellular functions and phenotype. It refers to covalent attachment of a methyl group to the C5 position of cytosine residue in CpG dinucleotide sequences preferentially located at the 5′ promoter region of human genes forming CpG islands. Methylation at cytosines, other than those in CpGs, occurs in undifferentiated cells and is crucial for gene regulation in embryonic stem cells [7]. CpG methylation plays an essential role in transcriptional gene silencing by restricting the expression of tissue-specific genes during development and differentiation, and is also involved in X chromosome inactivation in females, DNA imprinting, and transcriptional repression of highly repeated genome sequences. The donor methyl groups are supplied by S-adenosylmethionine (SAM) to form 5-methylcytosine (m5C). Methylation in CpGs suppresses transcription by either directly blocking DNA recognition and access at specific transcriptional factor binding sites or by recruitment of methyl-binding domain proteins (MBDs). For example, methyl-CpG binding protein 2 (MeCP2), a member of the MBD family, binds to methyl CpG recruiting histone-modifying proteins, such as histone deacetylases (HDAC). This leads to histone deacetylation, promoting chromatin condensation, and subsequent transcription repression [8]. CpG methylation is a post-replicative process and is mediated by DNA methyltransferase enzymes (DNMTs). DNA methyltransferase 3 alpha (DNMT3A) and DNA methyltransferase 3 beta (DNMT3B) are involved in *de novo* methylation during embryogenesis, while DNA methyltransferase 1 (DNMT1) preferentially methylates hemimethylated DNA during replication and is responsible for maintaining cellular CpG methylation status. As opposed to DNA methylation, DNA demethylation can recover transcriptionally repressed genes by the action of Ten-eleven translocation (TET) methylcytosine dioxygenases. The precise balance between methylation and demethylation of genome regulates the dynamic gene expression in cells and sustains homeostasis.

2.2 Posttranslational histone modifications (PTMs)

Within chromatin, DNA undergoes intricate packaging, forming a highly condensed structure wrapped around histone octamers. This arrangement results in the formation of nucleosomes, which gives the characteristic "beads on a string" appearance and can effectively regulate DNA accessibility. Each histone octamer is composed of a tetramer of two copies of histone 2A (H2A) and two copies of histone 2B (H2B), flanked by dimers of histone 3 (H3) and histone 4 (H4). The histone proteins feature a globular C-terminal domain and an extended N-terminal tail, which are susceptible to various PTMs. These include methylation of lysine or arginine residues, phosphorylation of serine or threonine, acetylation and deacetylation of lysines, and ubiquitylation and sumoylation of lysines. Acetylation and methylation of lysine residues on H3 and H4 are the most extensively studied PTMs. Histone acetylation is governed by the "charge neutralization model," wherein the positive charge of lysine residues on H3/H4 promotes tight DNA packaging with histones. Acetylation disrupts the tight configuration, allowing access for transcription factors, and thus facilitating transcription. Enzymes, such as histone acetyltransferases (HATs) and histone deacetylases (HDACs), regulate the addition and removal of acetyl groups. Unlike acetylation, histone methylation may have a different effect on targeted residues. For example, methylation at H3K4/36/79 generally activate transcription, while methylation at H3K9/27 and H4K20 is considered repressive [9]. Various histone methyltransferases (HMTs) catalyze these modifications, while removal of methyl groups from those marks is catalyzed by histone demethylases (HDMTs). Variations in the combinations of histone modifications, referred to as a "histone code," may regulate chromatin structure and transcriptional status [10]. The concept of a "histone code" significantly expands the informational capacity of the genetic code. Different histone variations can act synergistically or antagonistically in order to modulate the affinities of chromatin-associated proteins. This, in turn, regulates the dynamic transitions between transcriptionally active or transcriptionally inactive chromatin states. Overall, histone modifications play an important regulatory role bringing about different downstream events through the dynamic regulation of chromatin structure.

2.3 Noncoding RNAs (ncRNAs)

Noncoding RNAs have a regulatory function and are mainly categorized into long ncRNAs (lncRNAs) and small ncRNAs (sncRNAs). LncRNAs are a diverse family that consists of long transcripts from different genomic regions and are shown to play an essential role in X-chromosome inactivation and genomic imprinting. Their gene silencing effect is partly due to their recruitment of remodeling complexes, which foster histone methylation [11]. SncRNAs are also implicated in modulation of gene transcriptional silencing. These include microRNAs (miRNAs), small inhibitory RNAs (siRNAs), and piwi-interacting RNA (piRNA). While all classes mediate epigenetic modifications, piRNAs notably repress transposon expression through *de novo* DNA methylation [12]. Recent studies in mammals indicate implication of siRNAs and miRNAs in transcriptional gene silencing through the formation of epigenetic remodeling complexes, which promote DNA methylation, histone deacetylation, and methylation [13]. miRNAs can downregulate gene expression *via* complementary binding to the 3′ UTR of target mRNA. They play a crucial role as mediators in conferring robustness to biological processes by buffering small perturbations, thereby warranting homeostasis [14].

3. Environmental and lifestyle factors and the epigenome

The proper function of the organisms is a result of the delicate balance between the maintenance of the conserved nucleotide sequence, which facilitates the basic biological functions, and the dynamic changeability in the epigenome, which regulates gene expression, as a response to the constantly changing environment. This flexibility allows organisms to adapt to environmental shifts, and potentially "learn" from experience. The environmental impact on the regulation of gene expression plays a crucial role in reprogramming in early embryogenesis and development. During these stages, different sets of genes are epigenetically activated or deactivated, thus facilitating proper functioning of the organism through orchestrated events responsive to the environmental input. However, environmental factors, which affect gene expression networks, may disrupt the normal regulatory processes, potentially leaving long-lasting effects, and may even contribute to diseased outcomes. Many environmental and lifestyle factors were shown to epigenetically alter gene regulation and expression (**Figure 2**), and some of their known effects are discussed below.

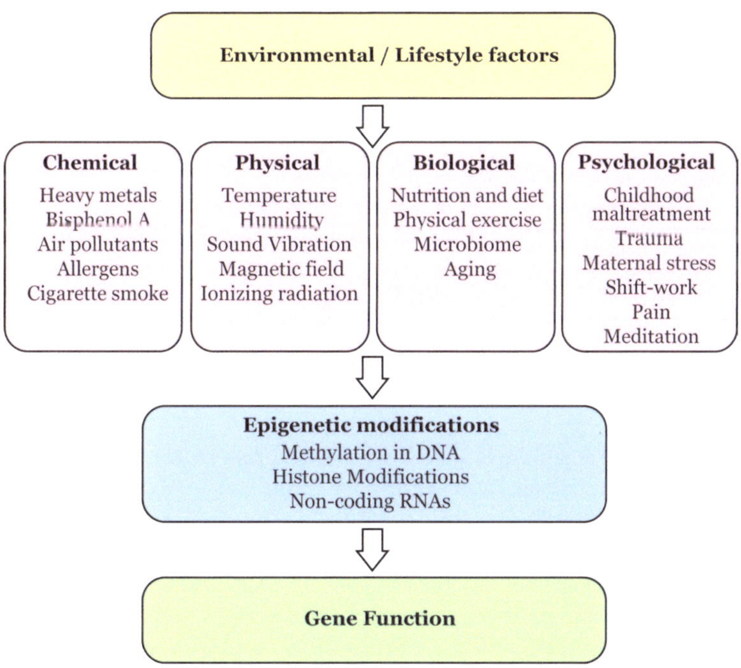

Figure 2.
Environment-epigenome interactions. Environmental and lifestyle factors, including chemical, physical, biological, and phycological, may cause changes in the epigenome, and thus can affect gene regulation and function by activating or silencing of genes.

3.1 Chemical factors

3.1.1 Heavy metals

Heavy metals, such as arsenic [15], cadmium [16], nickel [17], and lead [18], are common environmental pollutants that are able to impact DNA methylation, histone acetylation, and miRNA expression. Exposure to heavy metals in humans has been linked to a number of diseases, such as neurological disorders, cardiovascular conditions, central nervous system neuropathies, autoimmune diseases, and cancer and was shown to cause genotoxic and immunotoxic effects.

3.1.2 Bisphenol A (BPA)

Adverse consequences to the epigenome have also been demonstrated for another environmental chemical, bisphenol A (BPA), a common industrial plasticizer [19]. In mice, periconceptional exposure to BPA was shown to decrease the level of methylation in the IAP retrotransposon located upstream of the *Agouti* gene causing a change in the coat color distribution [20]. Mice with hypomethylation in this locus developed obesity, diabetes, and cancer at increased rates. However, the observed hypomethylating effect of BPA was reversed by maternal dietary supplementation with methyl donors, such as folic acid and the phytoestrogen genistein [21].

3.1.3 Air pollutants

Exposure to ambient air pollutants correlates with global genomic DNA methylation [22], increased H3K4 demethylation and H3K9 acetylation [23], modified expression of miR-21 and miR-222 [24], and has been linked to cardiovascular and respiratory diseases.

3.1.4 Allergens

Allergen exposure was reported to lead to deacetylation of histone proteins, hypermethylation of DNA, and changes in the levels of miRNA [25]. A genome-wide analysis demonstrated clear differential DNA methylation patterns in patients with seasonal allergic rhinitis [26].

3.1.5 Cigarette smoke

Exposure to cigarette smoke is a well-established risk factor for chronic obstructive pulmonary disease, cardiovascular diseases, and cancer. Alteration in DNA methylation at multiple CpG sites induced by cigarette smoke was reported in different populations, including Europeans [27], African Americans [28], and Chinese [29]. Moreover, whole-genome bisulfite sequencing has revealed differential CpGs methylation in cord blood of newborns exposed to prenatal maternal smoking [30]. Additionally, cigarette smoke exposure causes dose- and time-dependent histone alterations *in vitro,* which correlate with decreased DNMT genes expression [31], and differential expression of a number of miRNAs [32].

3.2 Physical factors

3.2.1 Temperature and humidity

Temperature extremes increase the risk for heatstroke, hyperthermia, or hypothermia and can worsen chronic conditions such as cardiovascular disease, respiratory disease, and diabetes. Studies have demonstrated an association between ambient temperature and relative humidity, LINE-1 and Alu methylation levels, and differential global DNA methylation *in vitro* upon heat and cold stress [33].

3.2.2 Sound vibration

Recently, it became apparent that sound vibration can induce physiological changes in plants mediated by epigenetic mechanisms as increased H3K27me3 in the promoter regions of defense-related genes in *Arabidopsis thaliana,* leading to immune activation against *Ralstonia solanacearum* [34].

3.2.3 Low-frequency magnetic fields

A few publications provided evidence that extremely low-frequency magnetic field exposure is related to increased global DNA methylation and aberrant site-specific DNA methylation [35], increased H3K9 acetylation [36], and altered miRNA expression [37].

3.2.4 Ionizing radiation

Ionizing radiation was also shown to cause epigenetic modifications, including global and gene-specific DNA methylation, histone modifications, and modulation of miRNA expression [38].

3.3 Biological factors

3.3.1 Nutrition and diet

Nutrition has been attributed epigenetic roles both in physiological and pathologic processes [39]. Folate deficiency, during conception and periconception, is related with several birth defects, including neural tube defects and congenital heart defects; however, application of folic acid periconceptionally can reduce birth defect frequency. The underlying mechanisms involve changes in the methylation of insulin-like growth factor 2 gene differentially methylation region (IGF2 DMR) [40]. Dietary choline, supplied prenatally or postnatally, leads to long-term enhancement of memory in rodents while choline deprivation during pregnancy decreases memory capacity in the offspring. A decrease in global DNA methylation and gene-specific DNA methylation of Cdkn3, which corresponded to increased expression of the encoded Kap protein, was reported in fetal brain from mothers fed a choline-deficient diet in mice [41]. Additionally, choline deficiency decreases H3K9me1 and H3K9me2 in murine fetal hippocampus and in cultured neural progenitor cells [42]. Decreased mean PPARα promoter methylation was found in the offspring of rats fed with a protein-restricted diet during pregnancy [43]. Alcohol consumption has been proven to cause global DNA hypomethylation and increased H3K43me in autopsy brain samples of patients with alcohol dependence [44]. Exposure to ethanol *in utero* can affect the epigenome of the developing mouse embryo causing changes in the phenotype [45].

3.3.2 Physical exercise

In addition to nutrition, physical exercise can significantly influence gene expression causing changes into the epigenome. A large number of differentially expressed genes were identified involved in metabolisms and mitochondrial biogenesis in skeletal muscle during recovery from endurance exercise [46]. The underlying mechanisms include increase in global leukocyte methylation [47] and global H3K36 acetylation [48] showing that exercise can induce chromatin remodeling associated with enhanced transcription.

3.3.3 Microbiota

Variations in the gut microbiota are related to many pathological conditions including intestinal and metabolic disorders, which can be mediated by microbiota-sensitive epigenetic mechanisms [49].

3.3.4 Aging

A role of epigenetic mechanisms in the process of aging and aging-related diseases was also established. Numerous studies on human and mouse tissues or cell cultures revealed that global DNA methylation generally decreases with age [50]. In addition, global changes in H3K9me3, H4K20me3, H3K27me3, and H3K9ac, and up- and downregulation of miRNAs in older individuals were also established [50]. Certain epigenetic modifications accumulate or change predictably with age providing a molecular signature that can be used to measure the aging process at a cellular level referred to as epigenetic clocks [51]. Epigenetic clocks are designed to estimate an individual's biological age rather than their chronological age. One of the most well-known epigenetic clocks is the Horvath Clock, which utilizes DNA methylation patterns at 353 specific CpG sites across the genome.

3.4 Psychological factors

3.4.1 Childhood maltreatment

A hundred of empirical studies explored the relation between childhood maltreatment and DNA methylation of candidate genes both in children and adults [52]. The vast majority of these investigate the methylation status of genes involved in the regulation of glucocorticoid signaling showing hypermethylation of NR3C1, hypomethylation of FKBP5, and differentially methylated CpG sites in children with a history of maltreatment [52].

3.4.2 Trauma

Exposure to trauma can also alter stress response mechanisms. In post-traumatic stress disorder (PTSD), dysregulation of hypothalamic-pituitary-adrenal (HPA) axis has been observed, which alters the response to cortisol feedback *via* differential methylation signatures [53].

3.4.3 Maternal stress

Maternal psychosocial stress experiences during pregnancy can permanently alter the function of the HPA axis causing site-specific CpG methylation in exposed individuals [54].

3.4.4 Shift-working

Shift-working occupations have been linked to increased risk of age-related diseases and were associated with epigenetic age [55]. The authors found that working more than 10 years of night shift work was significantly associated with epigenetic age acceleration. Additionally, differentially methylated CpG sites were associated with shift working, including the ZFHX3 gene, which is involved in circadian rhythm [55].

3.4.5 Chronic pain

Chronic pain can induce epigenetic modifications as well, including reduction in H3K27me3 levels at the Mcp-3 gene promoter [56], decrease in global DNA methylation [57], and increase in miR-155 and miR-223 expression [58] in prefrontal cortex in murine models.

3.4.6 Meditation

A few studies indicated that meditation can induce changes in the epigenome such as decrease in expression levels of HDAC2, HDAC3, and HDAC9 and alterations in global modification of H4ac and H3K4me3 predicting a better cortisol recovery after a test of acute psychosocial stress [59]. In meditators, the epigenetic aging rate was significantly decreased, which correlated with the number of years of practice [60].

4. Epigenetics and disease

Epigenetics was attributed two primary roles: one in normal development, guiding major biological processes such as reprogramming in early embryogenesis, and the other in disease, where epigenetic changes can contribute to certain pathological phenotypes. A great variety of epigenetic alterations have been found in a vast number of human diseases prompting for abnormal transcription activation or repression. Among these, cancer epigenome is most well-studied. Various epigenetic changes were reported in cancers of the breast, lungs, prostate, colorectum, ovaries, bladder, pancreas, gastric cancer, leukemia, and others [61–64]. The epigenetic component in tumorigenesis is characterized by abnormal patterns both in global DNA methylation and in local CpG methylation of target genes, disrupted patterns of PTMs, changes in chromatin composition and remodeling, and altered expression state of chromatin-modifying enzymes. A growing number of studies have attributed roles of miRNAs in almost all cancer types as well. Modifications in the epigenome take part in both cancer initiation and progression *via* silencing of tumor suppressor genes and activation of oncogenes and can predispose to genetic alterations through inactivation of DNA-repair genes.

Epigenetic modifications have also been associated with cardiovascular diseases such as coronary heart disease, acute myocardial infarction, heart failure, vascular calcification, and hypertension [65]. Aberrant DNA methylation patterns, histone modifications, and noncoding RNA regulation were shown to impact the function of cardiovascular disease-related genes and their expression levels, thus affecting cardiovascular disease progression.

A growing body of evidence attributes a role of epigenetics in a number of neurological (Alzheimer's, Parkinson's, and Huntington's diseases) and psychiatric disorders (depression, schizophrenia, bipolar disorder, autism spectrum disorders, and substance use disorders) and their co-occurrence, including dysregulation in DNA methylation and histone modifications resulting in disease phenotypes [66, 67].

All three types of epigenetic alterations, DNA methylation, histone modifications, and noncoding RNAs, are shown to be involved in the etiology of human autoimmune diseases, including systemic lupus erythematosus, rheumatoid arthritis, systemic sclerosis, Sjogren's syndrome, and autoimmune thyroid diseases [68].

A profound epigenetic component is described in the underlying mechanisms of metabolic diseases, such as obesity, type 2 diabetes, nonalcoholic fatty liver disease, osteoporosis, gout, and hyper- and hypothyroidism [69].

In a number of human disorders of genomic imprinting, such as Prader-Willi syndrome, Angelman syndrome, Beckwith–Wiedemann syndrome (BWS), pseudohypoparathyroidism (PHP), and Silver–Russell syndrome (SRS), "epimutations" leading to loss of gene expression were found, adding to the knowledge of how epigenetic defects lead to disease phenotypes [70].

The relationship between the genome and epigenome has extended our comprehension of the underlying molecular events that lead to human diseases. These could be either inherited or *de novo*, both genetic or epigenetic, and most notably, some might be influenced by the environment. Compared to genetic, epigenetic diseases display higher variability and heterogeneity, which can partially be explained by the distinctive characteristics of epigenetic modifications, such as potential reversibility, long-lasting effects, and responsiveness toward endogenous or exogenous stimuli. We could anticipate even greater environmental influence and a more substantial epigenetic contribution in both disease initiation and progression, considering that no cell repair mechanisms with regard to epimutations are thus far known. The study of epigenetics will allow us to better understand the relationship between environment, the changes in the epigenome, gene expression modulation, and disease.

The recognition of the role of epigenetics in the pathogenesis of diseases may justify why many therapeutic approaches in the past failed to achieve the anticipated outcomes. A deeper comprehension of the epigenetic mechanisms underlying human disorders is needed, and these hold promise for new therapeutic advancements. A breakthrough in the field of epigenetics and diseases is the approval of several epigenetic therapies (epidrugs) for cancer treatment [71]. The first approved DNMT inhibitor (DNMTi) primarily treats myelodysplastic syndrome by inhibiting DNA methylation, particularly targeting DNMT1 enzymes. The majority of approved compounds are HDAC inhibitors (HDACi), showing promise in selectivity and toxicity. Emerging therapies include miRNA and multidrug combinations which enhance cancer treatment and reduce drug resistance. Epigenetic therapies are continually assessed for cytotoxicity, pharmacological parameters, and mechanism of action in preclinical studies and in clinical trials.

5. Adaptation, homeostasis and allostasis

Over the course of millions of years, organisms have evolved characteristics, which allow them to fit exquisitely and operate optimally in their specific surroundings. However, these same traits may not be advantageous or beneficial in a different environmental context, and in some cases could even be detrimental to fitness. In view of the fact that no environment remains constant, even the most well-fitted organisms need be able to adapt to changes in order to survive. As a consequence, they have developed mechanisms designed to facilitate adaptation to changing environments. These allow them to cope with environmental challenges fostering resilience while faced with deviations from their usual operating conditions. In regard to this, the following types of responses to environmental changes may be undertaken by the organisms in pursuit of adaptation and survival:

Homeostasis: With homeostasis, the internal stability and balance within an organism are maintained relatively steady, regardless of external environmental fluctuations [72]. Homeostasis ensures that essential biological processes occur within a narrow range of optimal conditions.

Allostasis: The term "allostasis" was introduced by Sterling and Eyer [73] and literally means "maintaining stability through change." Allostasis refers to the adaptive process in response to acute environmental challenges [74]. While allostasis may appear similar to homeostasis, it emphasizes the flexible adaptation to dynamic environments or stressful circumstances. Unlike homeostasis, which seeks to maintain stability within a narrow range and minimize variability, allostasis recognizes that the optimal internal state may vary depending on situational demands. In allostasis, having greater variability is considered advantageous because it signifies the capacity of the internal settings to meet specific challenges posed by the environment in order to adapt and support the body's overall system [75]. When allostatic adaptive systems are activated and deactivated efficiently, "the body is able to cope effectively with challenges that it might not otherwise survive" [76].

Allostatic load: There are situations however where allostatic systems may be excessively stimulated or not functioning properly, and this state is referred to as "allostatic load" or the "cost of adaptation" [77]. "Allostatic load" describes the price that the body pays when it is compelled to adapt to challenging stressful conditions both physical and psychosocial. It indicates an excessive amount of stress or the inefficient functioning of the stress response systems, which should be activated during stress and then deactivated once the stressor subsides. When individuals experience repeated or chronic stressors, their bodies continuously activate the stress response. While the stress response is essential for coping with acute stressors, prolonged or repeated activation lacking adequate recovery can result in an accumulation of physiological dysregulation. Over extended periods of time, allostatic load can lead to the development of diseases [78]. McEwen distinguishes between the following types of allostatic load: repeated activation of allostatic systems that gradually lead to allostasis over time, failure to shut off allostatic activity after repeated stress resulting in failure to adapt, and insufficient primary adaptation mechanisms leading to the activation of compensatory mechanisms [77].

6. Epigenetic disease adaptational model (EDAM)

We will now explore the epigenetic disease in terms of environmental stress, epigenetic modification, and adaptative efficiency. By epigenetic disease, we will consider any pathological phenotype that is due to a change in gene expression in response to a stressful factor or a situation as a result of an epigenetic modification(s), which is either ontogenetic (occurring during the lifespan of an individual) or inheritable (epimutations), or both. Though genetic disease factors will not be considered here, in order to achieve simplicity, we will keep in mind that most diseases have a complex and multifactorial nature, and develop as a result of the interaction between both genetic and epigenetic determinants, that is. there is hardly a disease that is purely genetic or epigenetic. Moreover, genetic factors are involved not only in disease predisposition and progression but also may contribute to resilience, modulation of disease manifestation, immune response, disease recovery, or chronification. By epigenetic stress, referred below as "stress," we will assume any exogenous or endogenous, environmental or lifestyle factor of either physical, chemical, biological, or psychological nature that causes a shift in the homeostatic equilibrium *via* epigenetic modulation of gene expression. The roles of epigenetics in health and disease, apart from its role in cell differentiation and development, will be distinguished on the basis of the mode of response and the adaptive efficiency toward the stressful factor or situation as a body's attempts to maintain stability. Upon stress exposure, the following possible outcomes could be predicted depending on the nature, intensity and duration of the stress, the developmental period of stress exposure, and the efficiency of the epigenetic adaptational programs being triggered (**Figure 3**):

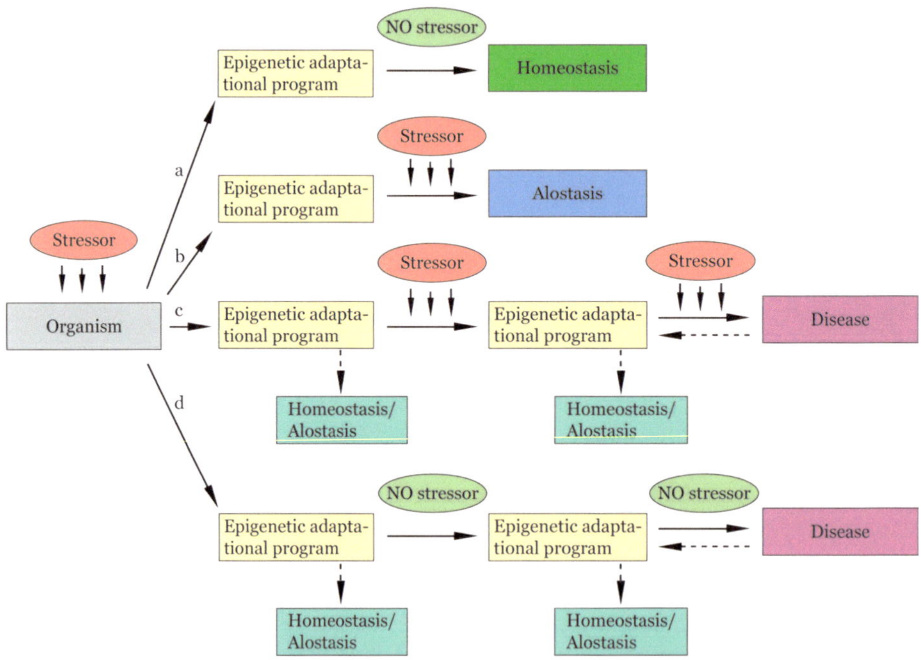

Figure 3.
Epigenetic disease adaptational model (EDAM). Upon stress exposure, epigenetic adaptational programs are triggered, which may have the following outcomes: (a) the epigenetic adaptational programs are adequate to the stressor/situation, and homeostasis is sustained, (b) the epigenetic adaptational programs are adequate to the stressor/situation and equilibrium is achieved via allostasis, (c) The epigenetic adaptational programs are not adequate to the stress nature, duration, intensity and/or period of action. The adaptation is not successful which is manifested in an epigenetic disease phenotype, and (d) the epigenetic adaptational programs are not adequate to the situation. Though the stress is switched off, the epigenetic adaptational programs are still operating. The stressful situation is wrongly considered the most probable situation and the stressful conditions are taken as "norm.". An epigenetic disease phenotype is manifested.

1. *Adaptation to the stress is successful and healthy equilibrium with environment is maintained or achieved.* This outcome will be attained when the epigenetic adaptational programs initiated during the stress response *are adequate* to the stress nature, duration, intensity, and/or period of action. In such a case, when the stress is turned off, the epigenetic adaptational programs will no longer be needed and will stop operating. Homeostasis will be sustained or allostasis will be reached (**Figure 3a** and **b**).

2. *Adaptation to stress is not successful and epigenetic disease programs are triggered.* In this case, the epigenetic adaptational programs *are not adequate* to the stress nature, duration, intensity, and/or period of action. Upon exposure to highly intense and continuous or repeated stress, notably in vulnerable developmental periods, in order to meet the challenges, the epigenetic adaptational programs triggered will continue operating in an attempt to maintain or achieve equilibrium. The failure of the organisms to adapt will be manifested in an epigenetic disease phenotype (**Figure 3c**). The epigenetic disease programs will, therefore, represent either inefficient epigenetic adaptational programs or additionally activated compensatory mechanisms, or both.

3. *Adaptation to stress is not anymore needed.* In circumstances such as these, the epigenetic adaptational program will not be adequate to the *situation*. This may occur in case the stress is already "turned off" but the epigenetic adaptational programs are still ongoing. The stressful situation is misjudged or the threat is being overrated. In such a case, the stressful situation is wrongly considered as *the most probable* situation, and the stressful conditions are taken as the "*normal*" (in the sense of "usual" or "becoming a standard") conditions. The still ongoing epigenetic adaptational programs are then outdated and needing a revision. An epigenetic disease phenotype will be manifested and/or sustained (**Figure 3d**).

7. Illustrating the EDAM model

Let us take two examples to illustrate the above postulations. Studies on Dutch Hunger survivors showed that maternal undernutrition has important effects on birth weights in newborns and health in later life, which are dependent on its timing during gestation [79]. Upon exposure to famine during the first trimester of pregnancy, the newborns were more likely to have normal birth weight though in later life they tended to display glucose intolerance and higher obesity rates than the general population, together with other health issues including coronary heart disease [80]. Moreover, all first-born offspring of such mothers (that were exposed to famine intrauterine) showed an increase in the average birth weight even though they themselves were never exposed to malnutrition during early development [81]. Studies on DNA methylation patterns in Dutch Hunger survivors have revealed alterations in key genes involved in metabolism [82, 83]. While correlation alone does not directly establish causation, the observed data are consistent with the assumption that undernutrition during early developmental stages alters the epigenetic code and expression profiles of key metabolic genes.

We can speculate that such dramatic metabolic stress, as is the huge reduction in nutrient supply during early gestation, can induce substantial alterations in the epigenetic processes within fetal cells. In response to the decreased nutrient supply, fetal cells will undergo metabolic adaptations in an attempt to sustain optimal fetal growth. The cells will modulate their gene expression patterns in order to counterbalance the nutritional deficiency. The epigenetic programming of fetal cells will allow optimal utilization of the limited nutritional resources. These alterations will be imprinted in the epigenome, setting the stage for future gene expression. Their biological purpose will be to attempt at adapting the developing organism to the stressful situation by maintaining optimal equilibrium with an environment that has been dramatically changed. Importantly, this programming will continue operating even after the cessation of the environmental stressor that prompted it. Moreover, these adaptational programs may even be passed into the offspring who may never in their lives encounter a similar stressful situation. Though transgenerational epigenetic inheritance presumably enables the transmission of beneficial survival solutions, it appears that at least some of these may not be relevant to the environmental context of next generations.

Notably, offspring whose mothers experienced malnutrition during the critical early stages of pregnancy, when the proper execution of the developmental programs is most crucial, exhibit an elevated susceptibility to adult obesity. During the initial stages of development, the fetus is particularly sensitive to stress-related responses controlled by epigenetic processes. In the early embryogenesis, significant changes occur in epigenetic markers due to the high level of cell division. It is likely that this vulnerability to stress responses during the early development may attempt to enable the most advantageous fitness to a surrounding considered most feasible in later life.

Another example comes from the studies on the long-term effects of early traumatic experience. Children who have experienced adversity or neglect in childhood are more likely to develop adult psychopathology, such as mood disorders and schizophrenia [84]. Individuals exposed to childhood trauma exhibit longstanding modifications of the HPA axis, a major neuroendocrine axis regulating homeostasis in mammals, and elevated cortisol metabolism. Upon stress, the HPA axis is activated, and the resultant increase in cortisol prepares the body to cope with the stressor. Under normal conditions, this system is controlled by a negative feedback loop, which restricts the stress response activity. This is dependent upon the expression of the glucocorticoid receptor (GR) gene, NR3C1, which is controlled by the level of promoter DNA methylation. In case the GR promoter is hypomethylated, the receptor is overexpressed and small cortisol amounts are needed to restrict stress response. Persons with a history of childhood abuse display increased methylation in the GR promoter [85], which prevents the NGFI-A transcription factor binding and causes low GR expression levels. The negative feedback loop is then compromised resulting in high stress hormone levels.

The maintenance of high cortisol levels in persons with early traumatic experience may be viewed as an adaptive mechanism utilized to enable readily available stress responses. It seems that this is achieved through epigenetic modulation of stress response genes. Even though these epigenetic adaptational programs have been triggered far away in time, they are still ongoing regardless of whether the stress is still present or not. We can assume that the traumatic situation is considered the *most feasible,* that is. “normal” situation. Maintaining the program active is then likely to manifest with different adult psychopathology observed in these cases.

8. Testing the EDAM model

The difficulty to test this model comes from the fact that most diseases are caused by multiple genetic and environmental factors. Furthermore, their effect is a result of factors interaction rather than of an individual influence. Different factors may act synergistically or antagonistically. Finally, we should take into consideration the possibility of occurrence of epigenetic changes, other than being adaptive, and the probable incidence of mutations in genes sequences, which can also contribute to the disease outcome. Nevertheless, a starting point for exploring the model can be the screening for epigenetic marks that can be related to a particular environmental or lifestyle factor, their possible significance for adaptation, and a further follow-up of how these are changed or sustained during pathology and recovery.

9. Conclusion

Organisms function in a fine balance with the environment, constantly adapting to changes, in order to maintain homeostasis or achieve allostasis. Upon stress, significant capacity for lasting adaptive plasticity is accomplished through epigenetic processes including methylation in DNA, PTMs, and ncRNAs. Cells undergo adaptations in an attempt to sustain optimal cellular functions. They modulate their gene expression patterns in order to counterbalance the stressor. The proposed EDAM model relies on the fine interplay between environmental stress, of either chemical, physical, biological or psychological nature, the response to it mediated through the epigenome, and how the failure to adapt may lead to epigenetic diseases. This may occur in at least two possible scenarios: first, when the epigenetic adaptational programs are not adequate to the stress nature, duration, intensity, and/or stage of action, and second, when the epigenetic adaptational programs are not adequate to the situation. In the last scenario, the stressful situation is wrongly considered the most feasible situation and the stressful conditions are taken as the "normal" conditions. Even though these adaptive programs may have been efficient in a past experience, their exact reproduction may be dysfunctional if not consistent with the current circumstances.

At least several questions rise from the proposed perspective: Are these not anymore advantageous programs editable? Have organisms evolved mechanisms to update the operating epigenetic adaptational programs with regard to the present context? In which cases is the stressful situation further considered a "norm" and how to counteract this? Are there set points at which: the epigenetic adaptational program turns into a disease program; the disease program can be brought back to health; and the disease program cannot be anymore reversed? What regulates the balance between these? How to monitor, and what strategies to use in order to manage the epigenetic burden that comes from the environment? How to target the modulation of the epigenome toward healthier states during life span and across generations?

The EDAM model adds a new perspective to understanding how failure to adapt to environmental stressors may lead to epigenetic diseases. Deeper understanding of the epigenetic bases of diseases has numerous potential applications. Some of these include (1) disease diagnosis and prognosis—epigenetic markers can serve as diagnostic tools for identifying diseases and predicting the course of the condition, (2) personalized treatment—allows for the development of targeted therapies based on an individual's unique epigenetic profile, (3) therapeutic interventions—development of new epidrugs aimed at reversing or modifying specific epigenetic modifications, and (4) environmental and lifestyle interventions—possibility of modifying epigenetic marks through changes in lifestyle, diet, or exposure to specific environmental factors.

Acknowledgements

The author is grateful to the National Science Fund of Bulgaria, Grant KP-06-H25/5 for the financial support of studies in the field of Epigenetics.

Conflict of interest

The author declares no conflict of interest.

Author details

Maria Emileva Krasteva
Bulgarian Academy of Sciences, Institute of Plant Physiology and Genetics, Sofia, Bulgaria

*Address all correspondence to: maria_krasteva@abv.bg

References

[1] Waddington CH. The epigenotype. Endeavour. 1942;**1**:18-20

[2] Wu C-t, Morris JR. Genes, genetics, and epigenetics: A correspondence. Science. 2001;**293**:1103-1105. DOI: 10.1126/science.293.5532.1103

[3] Turner B. Defining an epigenetic code. Nature Cell Biology. 2007;**9**:2-6. DOI: 10.1038/ncb0107-2

[4] Painter R, Osmond C, Gluckman P, Hanson M, Phillips D, Roseboom T. Transgenerational effects of prenatal exposure to the Dutch famine on neonatal adiposity and health in later life. BJOG: An International Journal of Obstetrics and Gynaecology. 2008;**115**:1243-1249. DOI: 10.1111/j.1471-0528.2008.01822.x

[5] Veenendaal MV, Painter RC, de Rooij SR, Bossuyt PM, van der Post JA, Gluckman PD, et al. Transgenerational effects of prenatal exposure to the 1944-45 Dutch famine. BJOG: An International Journal of Obstetrics and Gynaecology. 2013;**120**:548-554. DOI. 10.1111/1471-0528.12136

[6] Moore R, Kaletsky R, Murphy C. Piwi/PRG-1 Argonaute and TGF-ß mediate transgenerational learned pathogenic avoidance. Cell. 2019;**177**:1827-1841. DOI: 10.1016/j. cell.2019.05.024

[7] Lister R, Pelizzola M, Dowen RH, Hawkins RD, Hon G, Tonti-Filippini J, et al. Human DNA methylomes at base resolution show widespread epigenomic differences. Nature. 2009;**462**:315-322. DOI: 10.1038/nature08514

[8] Nan X, Ng HH, Johnson CA, Laherty CD, Turner BM, Eisenman RN, et al. Transcriptional repression by the methyl-CpG-binding protein MeCP2 involves a histone deacetylase complex. Nature. 1998;**393**:386-389. DOI: 10.1038/30764

[9] Wiles ET, Selker EU. H3K27 methylation: A promiscuous repressive chromatin mark. Current Opinion in Genetics & Development. 2017;**43**:31-37. DOI: 10.1016/j.gde.2016.11.001

[10] Jenuwein T, Allis CD. Translating the histone code. Science. 2001;**293**:1074-1080. DOI: 10.1126/science.1063127

[11] Mercer TR, Dinger ME, Mattick JS. Long non-coding RNAs: Insights into functions. Nature Reviews Genetics. 2009;**10**:155-159. DOI: 10.1038/nrg2521

[12] Ohnishi Y, Totoki Y, Toyoda A, Watanabe T, Yamamoto Y, Tokunaga K, et al. Small RNA class transition from siRNA/piRNA to miRNA during pre-implantation mouse development. Nucleic Acids Research. 2010;**38**(15): 5141-5151. DOI: 10.1093/nar/gkq229

[13] Morris KV. RNA-directed transcriptional gene silencing and activation in human cells. Oligonucleotides. 2009;**19**:299-306. DOI: 10.1089/oli.2009.0212

[14] Siciliano V, Garzilli I, Fracassi C, Criscuolo S, Ventre S, di Bernardo D. MiRNAs confer phenotypic robustness to gene networks by suppressing biological noise. Nature Communications. 2013;**4**:2364. DOI: 10.1038/ncomms3364

[15] Reichard JF, Schnekenburger M, Puga A. Long term low-dose arsenic exposure induces loss of DNA methylation. Biochemical and Biophysical Research Communications. 2007;**352**:188-192. DOI: 10.1016/j. bbrc.2006.11.001

[16] Takiguchi M, Achanzar WE, Qu W, Li G, Waalkes MP. Effects of cadmium on DNA-(cytosine-5) methyltransferase activity and DNA methylation status during cadmium-induced cellular transformation. Experimental Cell Research. 2003;**286**:355-365. DOI: 10.1016/s0014-4827(03)00062-4

[17] Lee YW, Klein CB, Kargacin B, Salnikow K, Kitahara J, Dowjat K, et al. Carcinogenic nickel silences gene expression by chromatin condensation and DNA methylation: A new model for epigenetic carcinogens. Molecular and Cellular Biology. 1995;**15**:2547-2557. DOI: 10.1128/MCB.15.5.2547

[18] Wright RO, Schwartz J, Wright RJ, Bollati V, Tarantini L, Park SK, et al. Biomarkers of lead exposure and DNA methylation within retrotransposons. Environmental Health Perspectives. 2010;**118**:790-795. DOI: 10.1289/ehp.0901429

[19] Singh S, Li SS. Epigenetic effects of environmental chemicals bisphenol A and phthalates. International Journal of Molecular Sciences. 2012;**13**:10143-10153. DOI: 10.3390/ijms130810143

[20] Morgan HD, Sutherland HE, Martin DIK, Whitelaw E. Epigenetic inheritance at the agouti locus in the mouse. Nature Genetics. 1999;**23**:314-318. DOI: 10.1038/15490

[21] Dolinoy DC, Huang D, Jirtle RL. Maternal nutrient supplementation counteracts bisphenol A-induced DNA hypomethylation in early development. Proceedings of the National Academy of Sciences of the United States of America. 2007;**104**:13056-13061. DOI: 10.1073/pnas.0703739104

[22] Tarantini L, Bonzini M, Apostoli P, Pegoraro V, Bollati V, Marinelli B, et al. Effects of particulate matter on genomic DNA methylation content and iNOS promoter methylation. Environmental Health Perspectives. 2009;**117**(2):217-222. DOI: 10.1289/ehp.11898

[23] Cantone L, Nordio F, Hou L, Apostoli P, Bonzini M, Tarantini L, et al. Inhalable metal-rich air particles and histone H3K4 dimethylation and H3K9 acetylation in a cross-sectional study of steel workers. Environmental Health Perspectives. 2011;**119**(7):964-969. DOI: 10.1289/ehp.1002955

[24] Bollati V, Marinelli B, Apostoli P, Bonzini M, Nordio F, Hoxha M, et al. Exposure to metal-rich particulate matter modifies the expression of candidate microRNAs in peripheral blood leukocytes. Environmental Health Perspectives. 2010;**118**(6):763-768. DOI: 10.1289/ehp.0901300

[25] Yang J, Zhong W, Xue K, Wang Z. Epigenetic changes: An emerging potential pharmacological target in allergic rhinitis. International Immunopharmacology. 2019;**71**:76-83. DOI: 10.1016/j.intimp.2019.03.004

[26] Nestor CE, Barrenäs F, Wang H, Lentini A, Zhang H, Bruhn S, et al. DNA methylation changes separate allergic patients from healthy controls and may reflect altered CD4+ T-cell population structure. PLoS Genetics. 2014;**10**(1):e1004059. DOI: 10.1371/journal.pgen.1004059

[27] Guida F, Sandanger TM, Castagné R, Campanella G, Polidoro S, Palli D, et al. Dynamics of smoking-induced genome-wide methylation changes with time since smoking cessation. Human Molecular Genetics. 2015;**24**(8):2349-2359. DOI: 10.1093/hmg/ddu751

[28] Dogan MV, Shields B, Cutrona C, Gao L, Gibbons FX, Simons R, et al. The effect of smoking on DNA methylation

of peripheral blood mononuclear cells from African American women. BMC Genomics. 2014;**15**:151. DOI: 10.1186/1471-2164-15-151

[29] Zhu X, Li J, Deng S, Yu K, Liu X, Deng Q, et al. Genome-wide analysis of DNA methylation and cigarette smoking in a Chinese population. Environmental Health Perspectives. 2016;**124**(7):966-973. DOI: 10.1289/ehp.1509834

[30] Howe CG, Zhou M, Wang X, Pittman GS, Thompson IJ, Campbell MR, et al. Associations between maternal tobacco smoke exposure and the cord blood CD4+ DNA methylome. Environmental Health Perspectives. 2019;**127**(4):047009. DOI: 10.1289/EHP3398

[31] Liu F, Killian JK, Yang M, Walker RL, Hong JA, Zhang M, et al. Epigenomic alterations and gene expression profiles in respiratory epithelia exposed to cigarette smoke condensate. Oncogene. 2010;**29**(25):3650-3664. DOI: 10.1038/onc.2010.129

[32] Schembri F, Sridhar S, Perdomo C, Gustafson AM, Zhang X, Ergun A, et al. MicroRNAs as modulators of smoking-induced gene expression changes in human airway epithelium. Proceedings of the National Academy of Sciences of the United States of America. 2009;**106**(7):2319-2324. DOI: 10.1073/pnas.0806383106

[33] Bind MA, Zanobetti A, Gasparrini A, Peters A, Coull B, Baccarelli A, et al. Effects of temperature and relative humidity on DNA methylation. Epidemiology. 2014;**25**(4):561-569. DOI: 10.1097/EDE.0000000000000120

[34] Jung J, Kim SK, Jung SH, Jeong MJ, Ryu CM. Sound vibration-triggered epigenetic modulation induces plant root immunity against Ralstonia solanacearum. Frontiers in Microbiology. 2020;**11**:1978. DOI: 10.3389/fmicb.2020.01978

[35] Liu Y, Liu WB, Liu KJ, Ao L, Li J, Zhong JL, et al. Effect of 50 Hz extremely low-frequency electromagnetic fields on the DNA methylation and DNA methyltransferases in mouse spermatocyte-derived cell line GC-2. BioMed Research International. 2015;**2015**:237183. DOI: 10.1155/2015/237183

[36] Leone L, Fusco S, Mastrodonato A, Piacentini R, Barbati SA, Zaffina S, et al. Epigenetic modulation of adult hippocampal neurogenesis by extremely low-frequency electromagnetic fields. Molecular Neurobiology. 2014;**49**:472-1486. DOI: 10.1007/s12035-014-8650-8

[37] Erdal ME, Yılmaz SG, Gürgül S, Uzun C, Derici D, Erdal N. miRNA expression profile is altered differentially in the rat brain compared to blood after experimental exposure to 50 Hz and 1 mT electromagnetic field. Progress in Biophysics and Molecular Biology. 2018;**132**:35-42. DOI: 10.1016/j.pbiomolbio.2017.08.001

[38] Belli M, Tabocchini MA. Ionizing radiation-induced epigenetic modifications and their relevance to radiation protection. International Journal of Molecular Sciences. 2020;**21**(17):5993. DOI: 10.3390/ijms21175993

[39] Choi SW, Friso S. Epigenetics: A new bridge between nutrition and health. Advances in Nutrition. 2010;**1**:8-16. DOI: 10.3945/an.110.1004

[40] Steegers-Theunissen RP, Obermann-Borst SA, Kremer D, Lindemans J, Siebel C, Steegers EA, et al. Periconceptional maternal folic acid use of 400 microg per day is related

to increased methylation of the IGF2 gene in the very young child. PLoS One. 2009;**4**:e7845. DOI: 10.1371/journal.pone.0007845

[41] Niculescu MD, Craciunescu CN, Zeisel SH. Dietary choline deficiency alters global and gene-specific DNA methylation in the developing hippocampus of mouse fetal brains. The FASEB Journal. 2006;**20**:43-49. DOI: 10.1096/fj.05-4707com

[42] Mehedint MG, Niculescu MD, Craciunescu CN, Zeisel SH. Choline deficiency alters global histone methylation and epigenetic marking at the Re1 site of the calbindin 1 gene. The FASEB Journal. 2010;**24**:184-195. DOI: 10.1096/fj.09-140145

[43] Lillycrop KA, Phillips ES, Torrens C, Hanson MA, Jackson AA, Burdge GC. Feeding pregnant rats a protein-restricted diet persistently alters the methylation of specific cytosines in the hepatic PPAR alpha promoter of the offspring. The British Journal of Nutrition. 2008;**100**(2):278-282. DOI: 10.1017/S0007114507894438

[44] Ponomarev I, Wang S, Zhang L, Adron Harris R, Dayne MR. Gene coexpression networks in human brain identify epigenetic modifications in alcohol dependence. The Journal of Neuroscience. 2012;**32**(5):1884-1897. DOI: 0.1523/JNEUROSCI.3136-11.2012

[45] Kaminen-Ahola N, Ahola A, Maga M, Mallitt KA, Fahey P, Cox TC, et al. Maternal ethanol consumption alters the epigenotype and the phenotype of offspring in a mouse model. PLoS Genetics. 2010;**6**(1):e1000811. DOI: 10.1371/journal.pgen.1000811

[46] Mahoney DJ, Parise G, Melov S, Safdar A, Tarnopolsky MA. Analysis of global mRNA expression in human skeletal muscle during recovery from endurance exercise. The FASEB Journal. 2005;**19**(11):1498-1500. DOI: 10.1096/fj.04-3149fje

[47] Zhang FF, Cardarelli R, Carroll J, Zhang S, Fulda KG, Gonzalez K, et al. Physical activity and global genomic DNA methylation in a cancer-free population. Epigenetics. 2011;**3**:293-299. DOI: 10.4161/epi.6.3.14378

[48] McGee SL, Fairlie E, Garnham AP, Hargreaves M. Exercise-induced histone modifications in human skeletal muscle. The Journal of Physiology. 2009;**587**:5951-5958. DOI: 10.1113/jphysiol.2009

[49] Woo V, Alenghat T. Epigenetic regulation by gut microbiota. Gut Microbes. 2022;**14**(1):2022407. DOI: 10.1080/19490976.2021.2022407

[50] Wang K, Liu H, Hu Q, Wang L, Liu J, Zheng Z, et al. Epigenetic regulation of aging: Implications for interventions of aging and diseases. Signal Transduction and Targeted Therapy. 2022;**7**(1):374. DOI: 10.1038/s41392-022-01211-8

[51] Oblak L, van der Zaag J, Higgins-Chen AT, Levine ME, Boks MP. A systematic review of biological, social and environmental factors associated with epigenetic clock acceleration. Ageing Research Reviews. 2021;**69**:101348. DOI: 10.1016/j.arr.2021.101348

[52] Parade SH, Huffhines L, Daniels TE, Stroud LR, Nugent NR, Tyrka AR. A systematic review of childhood maltreatment and DNA methylation: Candidate gene and epigenome-wide approaches. Translational Psychiatry. 2021;**11**(1):134. DOI: 10.1038/s41398-021-01207-y

[53] Howie H, Rijal CM, Ressler KJ. A review of epigenetic contributions to

post-traumatic stress disorder. Dialogues in Clinical Neuroscience. 2019;**21**(4):417-428. DOI: 10.31887/DCNS.2019.21.4/kressler

[54] Palma-Gudiel H, Córdova-Palomera A, Eixarch E, Deuschle M, Fañanás L. Maternal psychosocial stress during pregnancy alters the epigenetic signature of the glucocorticoid receptor gene promoter in their offspring: A meta-analysis. Epigenetics. 2015;**10**(10):893-902. DOI: 10.1080/15592294.2015.1088630

[55] White AJ, Kresovich JK, Xu Z, Sandler DP, Taylor JA. Shift work, DNA methylation and epigenetic age. International Journal of Epidemiology. 2019;**48**(5):1536-1544. DOI: 10.1093/ije/dyz027

[56] Imai S, Saeki M, Yanase M, Horiuchi H, Abe M, Narita M, et al. Change in microRNAs associated with neuronal adaptive responses in the nucleus accumbens under neuropathic pain. The Journal of Neuroscience. 2011;**31**(43):15294-15299. DOI: 10.1523/JNEUROSCI.0921-11.2011

[57] Tajerian M, Alvarado S, Millecamps M, Vachon P, Crosby C, Bushnell MC, et al. Peripheral nerve injury is associated with chronic, reversible changes in global DNA methylation in the mouse prefrontal cortex. PLoS One. 2013;**8**(1):e55259. DOI: 10.1371/journal.pone.0055259

[58] Descalzi G, Ikegami D, Ushijima T, Nestler EJ, Zachariou V, Narita M. Epigenetic mechanisms of chronic pain. Trends in Neurosciences. 2015;**38**(4):237-246. DOI: 10.1016/j.tins.2015.02.001

[59] Kaliman P. Epigenetics and meditation. Current Opinion in Psychology. 2019;**28**:76-80. DOI: 10.1016/j.copsyc.2018.11.010

[60] Chaix R, Alvarez-López MJ, Fagny M, Lemee L, Regnault B, Davidson RJ, et al. Epigenetic clock analysis in long-term meditators. Psychoneuroendocrinology. 2017;**85**:210-214. DOI: 10.1016/j.psyneuen.2017.08.016

[61] Baylin SB, Herman JG. DNA hypermethylation in tumorigenesis: Epigenetics joins genetics. Trends in Genetics. 2000;**16**:168-174. DOI: 10.1016/s0168-9525(99)01971-x

[62] Baylin SB, Jones PA. Epigenetic determinants of Cancer. Cold Spring Harbor Perspectives in Biology. 2016;**8**(9):a019505. DOI: 10.1101/cshperspect.a019505

[63] Portela A, Esteller M. Epigenetic modifications and human disease. Nature Biotechnology. 2010;**28**:1057-1068. DOI: 10.1038/nbt.1685

[64] Lu Y, Chan YT, Tan HY, Li S, Wang N, Feng Y. Epigenetic regulation in human cancer: The potential role of epi-drug in cancer therapy. Molecular Cancer. 2020;**19**(1):79. DOI: 10.1186/s12943-020-01197-3

[65] Shi Y, Zhang H, Huang S, Yin L, Wang F, Luo P, et al. Epigenetic regulation in cardiovascular disease: Mechanisms and advances in clinical trials. Signal Transduction and Targeted Therapy. 2022;**7**(1):200. DOI: 10.1038/s41392-022-01055-2

[66] Moosavi A, Motevalizadeh AA. Role of epigenetics in biology and human diseases. Iranian Biomedical Journal. 2016;**20**(5):246-258. DOI: 10.22045/ibj.2016.01

[67] Grezenko H, Ekhator C, Nwabugwu NU, Ganga H, Affaf M, Abdelaziz AM, et al. Epigenetics in neurological and psychiatric disorders: A comprehensive review

of current understanding and future perspectives. Cureus. 2023;**15**(8):e43960. DOI: 10.7759/cureus.43960

[68] Mazzone R, Zwergel C, Artico M, Taurone S, Ralli M, Greco A, et al. The emerging role of epigenetics in human autoimmune disorders. Clinical Epigenetics. 2019;**11**(1):34. DOI: 10.1186/s13148-019-0632-2

[69] Wu YL, Lin ZJ, Li CC, Lin X, Shan SK, Guo B, et al. Epigenetic regulation in metabolic diseases: Mechanisms and advances in clinical study. Signal Transduction and Targeted Therapy. 2023;**8**:98. DOI: 10.1038/s41392-023-01333-7

[70] Zoghbi HY, Beaudet al. Epigenetics and human disease. Cold Spring Harbor Perspectives in Biology. 2016;**8**(2):a019497. DOI: 10.1101/cshperspect.a019497

[71] Miranda Furtado CL, Dos Santos Luciano MC, Silva Santos RD, Furtado GP, Moraes MO, Pessoa C. Epidrugs: Targeting epigenetic marks in cancer treatment. Epigenetics. 2019;**14**(12):1164-1176. DOI: 10.1080/15592294.2019.1640546

[72] Cannon WB. The Wisdom of the Body. New York: W.W. Norton; 1932

[73] Sterling P, Eyer J. Allostasis: A new paradigm to explain arousal pathology. In: Fisher S, Reason J, editors. Handbook of Life Stress, Cognition, and Health. New York: John Wiley & Sons; 1988. pp. 629-649

[74] McEwen BS. Sex, stress and the hippocampus: Allostasis, allostatic load and the aging process. Neurobiology of Aging. 2002;**23**(5):921-939. DOI: 10.1016/s0197-4580(02)00027-1

[75] Carlson ED, Chamberlain RM. Allostatic load and health disparities: A theoretical orientation. Research in Nursing & Health. 2005;**28**(4):306-315. DOI: 10.1002/nur.20084

[76] McEwen BS. Protective and damaging effects of stress mediators: Central role of the brain. Dialogues in Clinical Neuroscience. 2006;**8**(4):367-381. DOI: 10.31887/DCNS.2006.8.4/bmcewen

[77] Mc Ewen BS. Stress, adaptation, and disease. Allostasis and allostatic load. Annals of the New York Academy of Sciences. 1998;**840**:33-44. DOI: 10.1111/j.1749-6632.1998.tb09546.x

[78] McEwen BS, Stellar E. Stress and the individual. Mechanisms leading to disease. Archives of Internal Medicine. 1993;**153**(18):2093-2101

[79] Lumey LH, Stein AD, Ravelli AC. Timing of prenatal starvation in women and birth weight in their first and second born offspring: The Dutch famine birth cohort study. European Journal of Obstetrics, Gynecology, and Reproductive Biology. 1995;**61**(1):23-30. DOI: 10.1016/0028-2243(95)02149-m

[80] Roseboom T, de Rooij S, Painter R. The Dutch famine and its long-term consequences for adult health. Early Human Development. 2006;**82**(8):485-491. DOI: 10.1016/j.earlhumdev.2006.07.001

[81] Lumey LH. Reproductive outcomes in women prenatally exposed to undernutrition: A review of findings from the Dutch famine birth cohort. The Proceedings of the Nutrition Society. 1998;**57**(1):129-135. DOI: 10.1079/pns19980019

[82] Tobi EW, Lumey LH, Talens RP, Kremer D, Putter H, Stein AD, et al. DNA methylation differences after exposure to prenatal famine are common

and timing- and sex-specific. Human Molecular Genetics. 2009;**18**(21):4046-4053. DOI: 10.1093/hmg/ddp353

[83] Heijmans BT, Tobi EW, Stein AD, Putter H, Blauw GJ, Susser ES, et al. Persistent epigenetic differences associated with prenatal exposure to famine in humans. Proceedings of the National Academy of Sciences of the United States of America. 2008;**105**(44):17046-17049. DOI: 10.1073/pnas.0806560105

[84] Devi F, Shahwan S, Teh WL, Sambasivam R, Zhang YJ, Lau YW, et al. The prevalence of childhood trauma in psychiatric outpatients. Annals of General Psychiatry. 2019;**18**:15. DOI: 10.1186/s12991-019-0239-1

[85] Shields AE, Wise LA, Ruiz-Narvaez EA, Seddighzadeh B, Byun HM, Cozier YC, et al. Childhood abuse, promoter methylation of leukocyte NR3C1 and the potential modifying effect of emotional support. Epigenomics. 2016;**8**(11):1507-1517. DOI: 10.2217/epi-2016-0074

Chapter 3

From Fluids to Forecasts: The Promise of Small Extracellular Vesicle miRNAs in Revolutionising Cancer Diagnostics

Sarwareddy Kartik Kumar and Manda Venkata Sasidhar

Abstract

Small extracellular vesicle (sEV) RNAs, particularly microRNAs (miRNAs), have emerged as pivotal biomarkers for cancer diagnosis and prognosis. Encapsulated within sEVs, these miRNAs reflect specific cellular characteristics and disease states, offering a window into cancers' molecular underpinnings. Notably, miRNAs, such as miR-7977, miR-98-3p, miR-620, and miR-17-5p in lung cancer and miR-373, miR-1246, miR-223-3p, and miR-21 in breast cancer, have been identified in sEVs extracted from various bodily fluids, including blood, urine, and saliva. Their remarkable stability and ease of isolation make them prime targets for non-invasive cancer detection strategies. The fold change of these miRNAs is intricately linked with cancer progression, metastasis, and therapeutic responses, underscoring their potential as diagnostic and prognostic markers. Traditional detection methods like quantitative reverse transcription-polymerase chain reaction (qRT-PCR) have been foundational; however, recent biosensing technologies, such as nanopore sequencing and microfluidic chips, offer enhanced sensitivity and specificity for detecting miRNAs in clinical samples. These innovative approaches refine the detection process and pave the way for real-time monitoring of disease progression and treatment efficacy. Overall, the collective evidence positions sEV miRNAs as robust indicators for cancer, signalling a shift towards personalised cancer care that emphasises early detection and tailored treatment strategies.

Keywords: extracellular vesicles, miRNA, mRNA, personalised medicine, RNA biomarkers

1. Introduction

Cancer remains a significant health challenge, necessitating early and adequate diagnostic measures. The advent of non-invasive cancer detection techniques heralds a new era of clinical diagnostics, enabling frequent monitoring of treatment effectiveness and facilitating adjustments to treatment plans for personalised care [1, 2]. Such advancements significantly enhance patient outcomes, allowing for early screening and diagnosis before the onset of symptoms and improving survival rates by treating cancers at stages when they are more responsive to therapy [3]. Despite progress in biomarker research aimed at alleviating the cancer burden, current diagnostic methods still grapple with issues of specificity, sensitivity, prolonged processing times, and invasiveness. The exploration of liquid biopsies marks a promising direction, yet the quest for cell-specific signatures with high reliability presents a formidable challenge [4]. Consequently, researchers increasingly focus on innovative approaches, especially developing biomarkers derived from minimally or non-invasive bodily fluids such as blood, urine, and saliva [4–6].

sEVs, such as exosomes, have emerged as critical players in this context. Originating from cellular endosomal compartments, these nanoscale membrane-bound vesicles (30–200 nm) reflect distinctive molecular signatures based on their cell of origin, carrying specific cargoes of RNAs, proteins, and lipids into the extracellular space [7, 8]. Contrary to earlier perceptions of sEVs as mere carriers of metabolic waste, ongoing research underscores their significant role in both physiological processes and pathological conditions [9]. The ability to non-invasively detect these vesicles in bodily fluids offers a window into cellular and disease processes, making sEVs a valuable tool in diagnosing, prognosis, and monitoring various cancers [8, 10].

The focus on cellular RNAs, particularly miRNAs, circRNAs, and lncRNAs, has intensified, given their roles in cancer pathophysiology [11–13]. The intersection of sEV cargo with miRNAs has garnered significant attention for its potential in cancer biomarker research. The transfer of sEV miRNAs can profoundly influence tumour progression, highlighting their importance in the disease molecular landscape [14, 15]. However, the field faces specific challenges, including technical difficulties in sEV miRNA detection and the need for standardised methodologies to ensure reliability and reproducibility across studies. Addressing these challenges is crucial for advancing the clinical application of sEV miRNAs as biomarkers. Recent studies exemplify the potential of sEV miRNAs in cancer diagnosis. For instance, research has demonstrated the efficacy of miR-21 encapsulated in EVs as a prognostic marker for non-small cell lung cancer, offering insights into tumour aggressiveness and patient survival outcomes [16]. Another study highlighted the role of sEVs miR-155 in breast cancer, correlating its levels with disease progression and response to treatment [17].

This chapter discusses the complex process of sEVs formation, selective packaging of miRNAs and their significance in cancer diagnosis. It provides a comprehensive overview of the biogenesis of sEVs from the plasma membrane to their release into the extracellular space, as well as the critical role played by various proteins in this process. The discussion also covers standard sEV isolation methods, such as ultracentrifugation, precipitation, and microfluidics, as well as recent advances in miRNA detection techniques including digital droplet PCR (ddPCR) and nanoflares. Further, this chapter also examines the advantages and drawbacks of these techniques and explores the analysis of sEV miRNA expression profiles in different types of cancer. This highlights the potential of sEV miRNAs as non-invasive biomarkers for early detection, diagnosis, and prognosis of cancer. Consequently, it provides valuable insights into tumour development, progression, and response to therapy.

2. sEVs biogenesis and miRNA packaging

sEVs are formed through a complex biogenesis process that unfolds in distinct stages. This process begins with the formation of endocytic vesicles from the plasma membrane, which then undergoes inward budding to form multivesicular bodies (MVBs) that house intraluminal vesicles (ILVs). Following their formation, MVBs can merge with lysosomes for degradation or fuse with the plasma membrane, releasing sEVs into the extracellular space (**Figure 1**). During these stages, various cytoplasmic biomolecules, including nucleic acids and proteins, are selectively incorporated into the lumen of EVs [18, 19].

Central to the biogenesis of sEVs is the action of the endosomal sorting complexes required for transport (ESCRTs), which are organised into four main complexes: ESCRT-0, ESCRT-I, ESCRT-II, and ESCRT-III. The process starts with ESCRT-0, which is responsible for gathering cargo molecules. ESCRT-I and ESCRT-II then contribute to the budding of the membrane, encapsulating the selected cargoes within. Following this, ESCRT-III is crucial in cutting the membrane to release ILVs packed with cargo into the MVB [18, 20, 21]. Accessory proteins, notably ALIX and TSG101, play essential roles in the efficient packaging of cargo and the overall biogenesis of EVs. ALIX aids in encapsulating cargo and forming vesicles by attracting ESCRT-III to the site, which is necessary for ILV formation. On the other hand, TSG101 is vital for forming MVBs triggered by EGF, a step critical for generating sEVs. These mechanisms ensure the selective packaging of molecular contents into sEVs, highlighting the sophisticated nature of exosome biogenesis and release [20, 22].

The process of sorting microRNAs (miRNAs) into sEVs involves a sophisticated interplay of RNA-binding and membrane proteins (**Figure 1**), as detailed in the 2020 review by Michael et al. [23]. Key RNA-binding proteins such as Heterogeneous nuclear ribonucleoprotein A2B1 (hnRNPA2B1), Argonaute 2, Y-Box Binding Protein 1, Major Vault Protein (MVP), and La Protein play crucial roles in this process. For instance, hnRNPA2B1 binds to miRNAs, aiding their incorporation into sEVs. Argonaute 2 transports miRNAs into sEVs through the KRAS-MEK-ERK signalling pathway. Similarly, Y-Box Binding Protein 1 facilitates miRNA loading into sEVs, while MVP and La Protein are responsible for the direct transfer of miR-193a into sEVs.

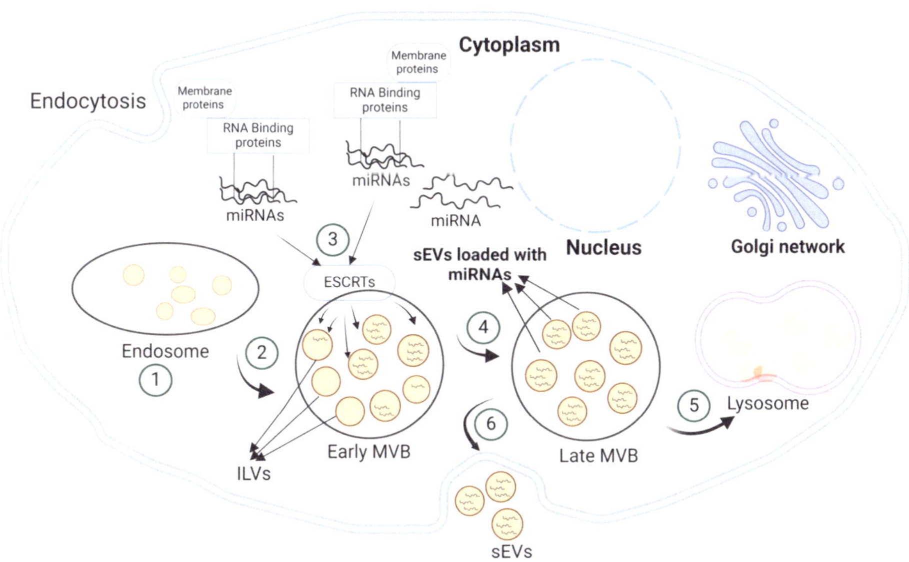

Figure 1.
Mechanism of sEV biogenesis and miRNA sorting. sEV biogenesis starts with formation of endosomes from the plasma membrane and is followed by development of MVB. Then, target miRNA molecules approach the MVB membrane for packing into sEVs. The sorting of miRNA into sEVs could be mediated by ESCRTs, RNA-binding proteins, and some of the membrane proteins. Afterwards, sEVs will be released into extracellular space by merging with lysosomes or fusing with plasma membrane.

Membrane proteins also contribute significantly to miRNA sorting. Caveolin-1 (Cav-1), for example, is essential in directing RNA-binding proteins to sEVs, especially under oxidative stress conditions. In such scenarios, Cav-1 influences the post-translational modifications of hnRNPA2B1, ensuring the selective incorporation of miRNAs into budding epithelial MVs [24]. Furthermore, the overexpression of Neural Sphingomyelinase 2 (nSMase2) has been shown to increase the expression of miRNAs in sEVs without altering the miRNA levels within cells [25]. Additionally, the overexpression of Vacuolar protein sorting-associated protein 4 (Vps4A) boosts the levels of sEV miR-27b-3p and miR-92a-3p, whereas inhibiting Vps4A decreases the levels of sEV-derived miR-92a and miR-150, as demonstrated in studies by Jin et al. and Charles et al., respectively [26, 27]. The complex process of directing miRNAs into sEVs showcases the synchronised actions of numerous proteins. Each of these proteins plays a specific role in accurately and methodically incorporating miRNAs into sEVs. This coordinated mechanism ensures that miRNAs can effectively participate in cellular communication and influence disease-related pathways [19].

In the context of cancer microenvironments, miRNA packaging into sEVs is influenced by additional, yet not fully understood, mechanisms, especially related to specific cancer conditions. Research by Diana et al. demonstrated that miR-10b is predominantly found in sEVs from wild-type cells, whereas miR-100 is more common in sEVs from cells with KRAS mutations [28]. Moreover, inhibiting NSMase resulted in an accumulation of miR-100 exclusively in the mutant cells, suggesting that the export of miRNAs can depend on the KRAS status. Another study by Sonia et al. showed that cancer-derived sEVs tend to accumulate the Dicer enzyme, facilitated by CD43, which is crucial for processing precursor miRNAs into their mature forms [29]. These discoveries highlight the intricate nature of miRNA sorting and processing within sEVs in cancer, pointing to novel diagnostic and therapeutic targets. Despite these insights, the exact reasons why miRNAs are sorted into sEVs in cancer remain debatable. The potential roles of this sorting range from simple elimination of cellular waste to participation in more complex biological processes [19, 30]. This uncertainty underscores the need for further research in sEV studies to fully understand the implications of miRNA sorting and its impact on tumour biology.

3. Isolation and characterisation of RNA-containing sEVs

Isolating and analysing RNA-containing sEVs are critical steps in unravelling their roles in biological processes and assessing their potential in cancer diagnostics. Researchers use various techniques to extract sEVs enriched with RNA from bodily fluids such as blood, saliva, and urine. Standard methods include ultracentrifugation, size exclusion chromatography, precipitation, microfluidics, immunoprecipitation targeting EV surface markers, and commercial isolation kits. As detailed in our previous review [31], each method varied with respect to the yield and purity of sEVs produced. In addition, every technique has advantages and limitations.

Ultracentrifugation is a technique that can handle large sample volumes but requires costly equipment. Precipitation methods are more cost-effective and can be used with various biological fluids and sample sizes; however, the risk of co-precipitating contaminants is a concern. Size exclusion chromatography (SEC) can be optimised for different sample volumes, but it requires more standardisation and can produce varying results depending on the material and sample being used. Immunoaffinity methods can capture sEVs with high purity and potential for

Cancer type	Molecules	Exosome origin	sEV isolation method	Expression status (increased/decreased)	Application	miRNA detection method	Ref
Lung	miR-7977	Serum	Commercial kit	Increased	Diagnosis	qRT-PCR	[32]
Lung	miR-98-3p	Serum	Commercial kit	Decreased	Diagnosis	qRT-PCR	[32]
Lung	miR-21-5p, -126-3p, and -140-5p	Serum	Ultracentrifugation	Increased	Early diagnosis	qRT-PCR	[33]
Lung	miR-146a-5p and miR-486-5p	Serum	Commercial kit	Increased	Early diagnosis	qRT-PCR	[34]
Lung	miR-620	Serum	Ultracentrifugation	Decreased	Diagnosis and prognosis	qRT-PCR	[35]
Lung	miR-20b-5p and miR-3187-5p	Serum	Ultracentrifugation	Decreased	Diagnosis	qRT-PCR	[36]
Lung	miR-17-5p	Serum	Commercial kit	Increased	Diagnosis	qRT-PCR	[37]
Lung	miR-21/Let-7a ratio	Serum	Commercial kit	Increased	Diagnosis	qRT-PCR	[38]
Lung	miR-451a	Plasma	Ultracentrifugation	Increased	Recurrence and prognosis	Microarray	[39]
Lung	miR-126	Serum	Ultracentrifugation	Decreased	Diagnosis and personalised therapeutic modality	qRT-PCR	[40]
Breast	miR-373	Serum	Commercial kit	Increased	Diagnosis	qRT-PCR	[41]
Breast	miR-1246	Plasma	Differential centrifugation	Increased	Diagnosis	Nucleic acid functionalised Au nanoflare probe	[42]
Breast	miR-223-3p	Plasma	Ultracentrifugation	Increased	Early diagnosis	qRT-PCR	[43]
Breast	miRNA-21-5p and miRNA-10b-5p	Serum	Commercial kit	Increased	Diagnosis and disease monitoring	qRT-PCR	[44]
Breast	miR-21	Plasma	Ultracentrifugation and commercial kit	Increased	Diagnosis	Dual-cycling nanoprobe	[45]

Cancer type	Molecules	Exosome origin	sEV isolation method	Expression status (increased/ decreased)	Application	miRNA detection method	Ref
Brain	miR-21	CSF	Ultracentrifugation	Increased	Diagnosis and tumour recurrence	qRT-PCR	[46]
Brain	miR-301a	Serum	Commercial kit	Increased	Diagnosis and prognosis	qRT-PCR	[47]
Brain	miR-210	Serum	Ultracentrifugation	Increased	Diagnosis and prognosis	qRT-PCR	[48]
Brain	miR-2276-5p	Plasma	Ultracentrifugation	Decreased	Diagnosis and prognosis	qRT-PCR	[49]
Colon	miR-139-3p	Plasma	Commercial kit	Decreased	Early diagnosis and metastasis	qRT-PCR	[50]
Colon	miR-377-3p and miR-381-3p	Serum	Ultracentrifugation	Decreased	Early diagnosis	qRT-PCR	[51]
Colon	miR-196b-5p	Serum	Commercial kit	Increased	Diagnosis	qRT-PCR	[52]
Prostate	miR-141	Serum	Commercial kit	Increased	Diagnosis	qRT-PCR	[53]
Prostate	MiR-30b-3p and miR-126-3p	Urine	Ultracentrifugation	Increased	Diagnosis	Microarray	[54]
Prostate	miR-20b-5p	Prostatic fluid	Commercial kit	Increased	Early diagnosis	qRT-PCR	[55]
Prostate	miR-181a-5p	Serum	Commercial kit	Increased	Diagnosis	Deep sequencing and Chip array	[56]
Ovarian	miR-200a-3p, miR-766-3p, miR-26a-5p, miR-142-3p, let-7d-5p, and miR-328-3p	Serum	Ultracentrifugation	Increased	Early diagnosis	qRT-PCR	[57]
Ovarian	miR-145 and miR-200c	Serum	Commercial kit	Increased	Preoperative diagnosis	qRT-PCR	[58]
Gastric	miR-21	Plasma	Ultracentrifugation	Increased	Recurrence	Microarray	[59]
Gastric	miR-92a	Plasma	Ultracentrifugation	Decreased	Recurrence and prognosis	Microarray	[59]

Cancer type	Molecules	Exosome origin	sEV isolation method	Expression status (increased/ decreased)	Application	miRNA detection method	Ref
HCC	miR-4661-5p	Serum	Commercial kit	Increased	Early diagnosis	qRT-PCR	[60]
HCC	miR-21	Serum	Commercial kit	Increased	Diagnosis	qRT-PCR	[61]
Thyroid	miR-29a	Serum	Commercial kit	Decreased	Diagnosis and prognosis	qRT-PCR	[62]
Bladder	miR-96-5p and miR-183-5p	Urine	Commercial kit	Increased	Diagnosis	qRT-PCR	[63]
Oral	miR-130a	Plasma	Commercial kit	Increased	Diagnosis and prognosis	qRT-PCR	[64]

Table 1.
sEV miRNA expression patterns across different cancer types.

subtyping, but they are only suitable for small sample volumes. Microfluidics-based isolation can yield high-purity sEVs, but it has limited sample capacity and the conditions may affect the stability of the vesicles. Commercial kits can be used for simplicity and to preserve the integrity of sEVs, but they are expensive and less suitable for diluted samples like urine. Therefore, choosing the appropriate method for efficient sEV isolation is essential based on the sample volume and type [31]. Previous studies have mainly used commercial kits and ultracentrifugation to isolate sEVs from serum, plasma, and urine (**Table 1**).

Following isolation, the characterisation of these RNA-containing sEVs employs a range of techniques. Nanoparticle tracking analysis (NTA) and transmission electron microscopy (TEM) are utilised to assess the EVs size, concentration, and structural details. Researchers estimate ratios such as proteins to particles, lipids to particles, or lipids to proteins for broader quantification. Techniques like Western blotting, ELISA, and RT-qPCR detect specific proteins and genes associated with EVs, serving as markers. Mass spectrometry further complements these methods by profiling the protein content of the EVs, offering more profound insights into their molecular composition [31]. Together, these characterisation techniques verify the quality and quantify the isolated RNA-containing sEVs, providing a thorough understanding of their potential for diagnostic applications.

4. Detection of sEV miRNA

Quantitative real-time PCR (qRT-PCR) is widely used to identify and quantify sEV miRNA expression (**Table 1**). Still, ddPCR enhances this quantification with superior sensitivity, reproducibility, and accuracy [65]. Additionally, innovative methods like electrochemical sensing and surface-enhanced Raman scattering (SERS) are showing promising results in terms of consistency and selectivity. For instance, Lipei et al. crafted a biosensor that combines electrochemical detection, ratiometric readout, and DNA structural transformation to sensitively detect EV miR-21, achieving a detection limit as low as 2.3 femtomolar (fM) [66]. This method stands out for its enhanced stability and reliability. Similarly, Xinyu et al. unveiled an ultra-sensitive electrochemical biosensor employing cascade catalytic hairpin assembly (CHA) and multilayered enzymes for detecting trace amounts of miRNA-21 in actual samples [67]. Yue et al. designed a microfluidic SERS sensor capable of detecting EV miRNA as low as 1 pmol/L, employing rolling circle amplification (RCA) and tyramine signal amplification (TSA) to boost sensitivity significantly [68]. In the realm of colorimetric detection, Yaokun et al. developed a copper-mediated strategy that uses DNAzyme signal amplification and visible light-triggered reactions for pinpointing miR-21 presence [69].

On the device front, Takao et al. presented a nanowire-anchored microfluidic device that efficiently isolates urine sEV-encapsulated miRNAs [70]. This device promises to enhance cancer diagnostics by facilitating rapid miRNA extraction from minimal urine volumes and is applicable to a wide range of cancers beyond just urological ones. Building on this, Xue et al. combined nanoflare technology with CHA amplification for in situ, extraction-free, and highly sensitive sEV miRNA analysis. Their clinical tests show potential for accurately distinguishing different cancer types with 99% accuracy from plasma samples [71]. Furthermore, Xuting et al. introduced a novel method for detecting sEV miR-1246 with high sensitivity by creating hybrids between sEVs and cationic liposomes, allowing for precise quantification of sEV miR-1246 [72]. Together, these advancements highlight significant progress in the field of sEV miRNA detection, offering improved sensitivity and potential for clinical application in disease diagnostics.

5. sEV miRNA as diagnostic tools in cancer

miRNAs are crucial for gene regulation in eukaryotic organisms, affecting a wide range of developmental and disease processes. These miRNAs can be found in body fluids like saliva, urine, and blood, maintaining their stability within EVs. The miRNAs within sEVs, which reflect those of the tumour cells they originate from, are emerging as valuable biomarkers for cancer due to their durability and unique expression profiles [18, 19]. Initial research, such as the study conducted by Guilherme in 2009, found that miRNA profiles from sEVs in peripheral circulation and those from tumour-derived sEVs were similar, but the average concentration of miRNAs was significantly different in control groups [73]. This was followed by studies demonstrating the feasibility of detecting sensitive prostate cancer markers in sEV RNA from small urine samples [74]. In 2010, Keiichi and colleagues spotlighted the significance of the let-7 miRNA family in identifying metastatic gastric cancer through sEVs [75]. These early findings laid the groundwork for using sEV RNA as a snapshot of the tumour's genetic landscape, facilitating miRNA analysis without the need for tissue samples. This approach is promising for screening people without symptoms and tracking disease recurrence, enhancing cancer diagnostics in recent years. The streamlined workflow for identifying sEV miRNA-based biomarkers in cancer diagnosis is illustrated in **Figure 2**.

In lung adenocarcinoma (LUAD) patients, increased levels of serum sEV miRNA ExomiR-7977 and reduced miR-98-3p highlight their potential as markers for diagnosis and staging accuracy [32]. Min and colleagues discovered elevated sEV miRNAs, such as ex-miR-21-5p, -126-3p, and -140-5p, suggesting these are precise, sensitive, and reliable markers for LUAD diagnosis [33]. Additionally, early-stage non-small cell lung cancer (NSCLC) showed significantly higher levels of serum sEV miR-146a-5p and miR-486-5p compared to benign conditions and healthy individuals, according to qRT-PCR results. The combination of serum and sEV miRNAs increased diagnostic sensitivity and specificity [34]. Recent breakthroughs in technology have brought about a novel biosensor that leverages nanoflare technology and catalysed hairpin assembly (CHA) amplification. This tool allows for direct, highly sensitive analysis of miRNAs within sEVs without the need for sample extraction. In clinical cohort, this method distinguished between breast, lung, liver, cervical, and colon cancers in 64 patients with an astonishing 99% accuracy, showcasing its precision in cancer diagnosis [71].

Research has identified a significant increase in hsa-miR-21-5p levels within breast cancer (BC) sEVs, making it possible to differentiate BC patients from healthy individuals with a high degree of accuracy (sensitivity of 86.7% and specificity of 93.3%, as per ROC analysis) [76]. Pre-therapy miRNA profiling of 435 BC patients revealed variations in expression across different subtypes, with miR-155 and miR-301 linked to predicting responses to treatment. Notably, the miRNA profile varied significantly between the overall BC cohort, those with HER2-positive BC, and patients with triple-negative BC [17]. A particular study found that elevated levels of sEV miR-373 were associated with triple-negative and more aggressive forms of BC, indicating its potential for diagnostic use [41]. Continuing research efforts include developing

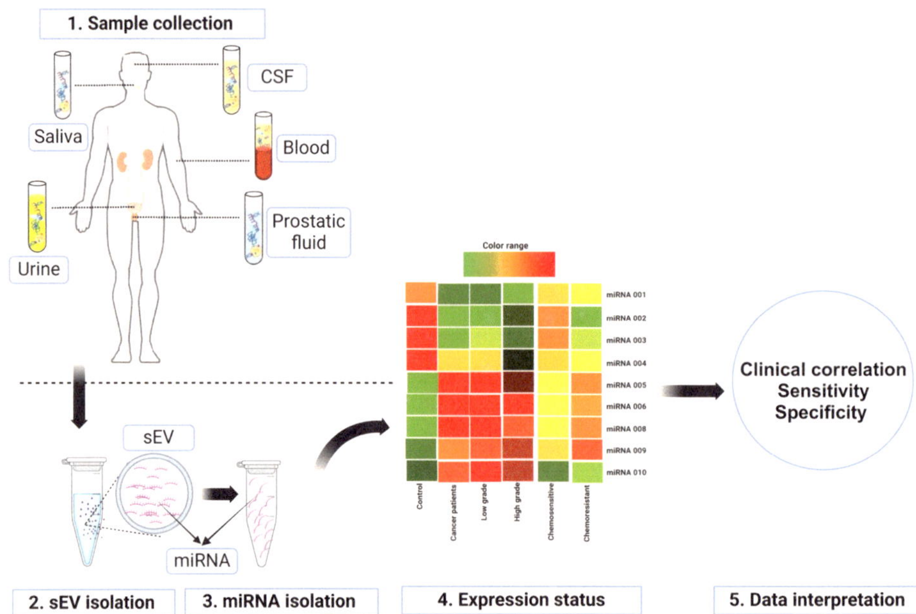

Figure 2.
Detection workflow of sEV miRNA-based biomarkers in cancer diagnosis. This figure presents a streamlined workflow for identifying miRNA biomarkers within sEVs for cancer diagnostics. The process begins with the collection of biofluid samples, including blood, urine, and saliva, which are rich sources of sEVs. Following collection, sEVs are meticulously isolated from these samples to retrieve their miRNA cargo. The extracted miRNAs are then subjected to qPCR for precise quantification and analysis of specific miRNA expression patterns associated with various cancer types. The final step involves evaluating the clinical relevance of these miRNA signatures by determining their correlation with the presence of cancer, its progression, and its response to treatment, alongside assessing the diagnostic sensitivity and specificity based on the gathered data.

methods for direct miRNA detection from exosomes in breast cancer cases, such as the introduction of an Au nanoflare probe by Leu et al. [77]. This probe, designed to target miR-1246 specifically, enters plasma sEVs and emits a fluorescent signal, offering a simple, accurate, and sensitive diagnostic approach.

In glioma, analysis of cerebrospinal fluid (CSF) from patients with recurrent disease revealed higher levels of sEV miR-21, suggesting its utility as a marker for diagnosis and prognosis [46]. This increase in EV miR-21 was found to correlate with tumour metastasis and recurrence. Within glioma tissues, miR-21 concentrations were associated with the tumour's grade and inversely correlated with patient survival rates. Experiments showing the suppression of miR-21 in glioma cells led to the upregulation of target genes, implicating its role in the progression of glioma. Additionally, increases in serum sEV miR-301a and miR-210 were observed in glioma patients, correlating with the severity and recurrence of the tumour [47, 48]. On the other hand, a decrease in plasma sEV miR-2276-5p was linked to poorer survival outcomes in glioma patients, identifying RAB13 as its target [49]. These discoveries underscore the significant potential of sEV miRNAs as biomarkers for the diagnosis and prognosis of glioma.

In colorectal cancer (CRC), the discovery of sEV miR-320d as a non-invasive marker has been pivotal in differentiating metastatic from non-metastatic cases, offering a clearer path for diagnosis and treatment strategies [78]. Additionally, miR-125a-3p and miR-122 found in plasma sEVs have been identified to not only aid in the early diagnosis of colon cancer but also serve as independent prognostic indicators, particularly for patients with liver metastasis [79, 80]. On the other hand, a decrease in sEV miR-139-3p levels in CRC patients, especially those with metastatic and submucosal involvement, has been noted as a potential marker for prognosis [50]. A group of sEV miRNAs, including miR-100 and miR-92a, has shown potential in distinguishing between chemotherapy-resistant and -sensitive CRC patients [81]. Bioinformatics analyses have further highlighted an sEV miRNA-mRNA network that plays a critical role in CRC, underlining the diagnostic importance of these circulating biomarkers [82].

In the realm of prostate cancer (PCa), serum sEV miR-141 has shown promise as a diagnostic biomarker, particularly noting its significant increase in cases of metastatic PCa compared to healthy individuals or those with benign prostatic hyperplasia (BPH) [53]. A study by Kyosuke et al. demonstrated the superiority of urine sEV samples in diagnosing PCa, with miR-30b-3p and miR-126-3p showing higher expression levels than traditional serum prostate-specific antigen (PSA) markers [54]. Further analysis by Manuel et al., using the International Society of Urological Pathology (ISUP) grading system, identified differentially expressed miRNAs that could help in the nuanced management of PCa under active surveillance, showing strong potential with AUCs ranging from 0.79 to 0.88 [83]. Expanding on this, Zhenquan et al. discovered plasma exosome-derived miRNAs, including hsa-miR-125a-3p, hsa-miR-330-3p, hsa-miR-339-5p, and has-miR-613, as potential markers for detecting bone metastasis in PCa patients, marking significant progress in the development of non-invasive diagnostic and prognostic tools for prostate cancer [84].

Research into sEV miRNAs as tools for diagnosing and prognosticating a wide array of cancers, including bladder, ovarian, gastric, hepatocellular, thyroid, oral, and oropharyngeal cancers, underscores their vast potential across a myriad of cancer types. This wide-ranging investigation highlights the critical role of sEV miRNAs in enhancing the accuracy of cancer diagnosis and improving patient prognoses. In the case of bladder cancer, the detection of elevated levels of specific urinary sEV miRNAs, such as miR-96-5p, miR-183-5p, miR-93-5p, and miR-516a-5p, has been linked to significant clinicopathological features, offering a new method for early detection [63, 85]. A study by Akira et al. revealed that a combination of six miRNAs isolated from serum sEVs of ovarian cancer patients, when used alongside the CA-125 marker, greatly improved the sensitivity and specificity of tests for distinguishing ovarian cancer patients from healthy individuals, and for identifying early-stage ovarian cancer from benign tumours [57]. Furthermore, Naruyoshi et al. identified plasma sEV miR-21 and miR-92a as independent markers for the early detection of gastric cancer [59]. Additionally, Yoshimasa et al. found that sEV miR-23b serves as a reliable indicator for the recurrence and prognosis of gastric cancer at various stages [86].

In hepatocellular carcinoma (HCC), the enrichment of miR-21 in serum sEVs offers a more sensitive detection method, as highlighted by Hongwei et al. [61]. The presence of elevated levels of miR-122, miR-148a, and miR-1246 in serum sEVs, in combination with alpha-fetoprotein, has been shown to enhance the diagnostic accuracy for early-stage HCC significantly [87]. Chen et al. reported that lower levels of serum sEV miR-34a are associated with poorer survival rates in HCC patients [88], suggesting that its combination with other biomarkers like alpha-fetoprotein could improve diagnostic effectiveness.

The role of serum sEV miRNAs in diagnosing and prognosticating papillary thyroid carcinoma (PTC) has also been elucidated in recent studies. For instance, decreased levels of miR-29a in PTC patients have been shown to differentiate them from healthy controls, with this downregulation correlating with more aggressive disease characteristics and poorer patient outcomes [62]. Moreover, circulating sEV miR-146b-5p and miR-222-3p have emerged as significant markers for detecting lymph node metastasis in PTC [89]. In oral squamous cell carcinoma, the diagnostic and prognostic value of both plasma and saliva sEV miRNAs, including miR-130a and miR-486-5p, has been demonstrated, with miR-486-5p showing a robust correlation with stage II of the disease [64, 90]. These discoveries collectively affirm the crucial role of sEV miRNAs as biomarkers for the diagnosis and prognosis of various cancers, offering promising avenues for non-invasive testing and tailored patient care. A comprehensive table summarising the expression patterns of different sEV miRNAs across various cancer types further illustrates their diagnostic and prognostic utility (**Table 1**).

6. EV RNA databases

In the fast-evolving field of sEV RNA research, several vital databases have become critical for researchers. These platforms enable the collection, access, and analysis of data on EV RNA, playing a crucial role in advancing our understanding of these nano-vesicles. ExoCarta is a standout resource that provides detailed information on the molecular contents of EVs, including mRNAs, miRNAs, proteins, and lipids. It compiles data from 286 studies covering a wide range of organisms, making it a rich source of information for researchers. This web-based platform also supports detailed functional analysis and interaction studies, and it actively encourages the EV community to contribute by identifying publications that might have been overlooked, thereby continuously expanding its database [91, 92]. EVpedia is another comprehensive database that offers an integrated view of sEVs, compiling data from 503 high-throughput studies, 1114 datasets, and over 722,551 molecules. It is designed to enable comparisons across different studies and is particularly useful for exploring the RNA content of EVs. Since 2010, there has been a notable increase in the volume of articles, especially those related to eukaryotic organisms, aiding in discovering biomarkers and potential therapeutic targets [93]. VESICLEpedia consolidates a wide array of information on sEVs and related particles like microvesicles and apoptotic bodies. It comprehensively examines EVs' various cargos, including lipids, metabolites, nucleic acids, and proteins. This repository is invaluable for researchers focused on the diagnostic and therapeutic applications of EV RNA in various diseases [94]. Together, these databases represent vital tools for the EV RNA research community, offering extensive data repositories that support the exploration of EV functions, the identification of disease biomarkers, and the development of novel therapeutic strategies.

In the focused area of EV RNA research, three specialised databases have been developed to meet the varied needs of the EV community. These resources are crucial in advancing our understanding of extracellular RNA (exRNA), providing data storage, access, and analysis platforms. exRNA Atlas, created by the exRNA Communication Consortium (ERCC), is a dedicated repository for exRNA data. It contains a wealth of sequencing and RT-qPCR data from a wide range of human and mouse biofluids. The database enables users to search and analyse exRNA profiles based on the type of assay and specific biofluids, aiding in the identification and study of exRNA related to different health conditions and diseases [95]. exoRBase offers a focused look at long RNAs within EV, covering messenger RNA (mRNA),

Database	Focus	Website link
ExoCarta	Exosomal mRNA, miRNAs, proteins, and lipids	http://www.exocarta.org/
EVpedia	EV mRNA, miRNAs, proteins, and lipids	https://evpedia.info/evpedia2_xe/
VESICLEpedia	EV mRNA, miRNAs, proteins, and lipids	http://microvesicles.org/
exRNA Atlas	Exosomal RNA	http://exrna-atlas.org/
exoRBase	Exosomal long RNA species: mRNAs circRNAs, and lncRNAs	http://www.exorbase.org/
miRandola	Non-coding RNA	http://mirandola.iit.cnr.it/

Table 2.
EV RNA databases and their focused molecules.

long non-coding RNA (lncRNA), and circular RNA (circRNA) derived from various human body fluids. This database integrates and visualises RNA expression profiles, highlighting changes in functional pathways and the heterogeneity of circulating EVs. With a primary focus on blood-derived samples, exoRBase is a valuable tool for in-depth studies and comparative analysis of EV RNA [96]. miRandola is a niche database that centres on miRNAs band and includes information on lncRNAs and circRNAs. It features a network visualisation of RNA-disease associations, compiled from the scientific literature, to illuminate the connections between specific RNAs and different tumours. This functionality is particularly beneficial for researching the roles of potential RNA biomarkers in cancer, offering insights into how these molecules interact with various diseases [97]. These databases (**Table 2**) collectively advance EV RNA research by providing centralised data deposition, sharing, and analysis platforms. Researchers can leverage these resources to delve into the complexities of EV RNA content and its relevance in diverse biological contexts. These are expected to evolve as the field progresses, accommodating new findings and technologies in EV RNA research, further catalysing discoveries and innovations in this rapidly expanding field.

7. Conclusions

In conclusion, studies on sEV RNAs in cancer research have indeed revealed a wealth of potential diagnostic and prognostic biomarkers. These discoveries offer profound insights into the underlying mechanisms of various cancers and pave the way for innovative therapeutic interventions. In particular, sEV miRNAs have garnered attention for their remarkable stability, specificity, and detectability in a multitude of bodily fluids, making them excellent candidates for biomarker discovery in cancer. Researchers have identified numerous sEV miRNA signatures that correlate with different types of cancer, disease stages, and prognoses, significantly enhancing our capacity to diagnose, monitor, and potentially predict disease outcomes. However, it is imperative to recognise that much of the current evidence is derived from studies with relatively small sample sizes. There is a pressing need for further validation studies involving larger cohorts to determine the clinical utility of these biomarkers conclusively. Additionally, there has been limited research into the dynamic changes of circulating sEV miRNAs before and after cancer treatment, which could offer invaluable insights into the effectiveness of therapeutic interventions.

The potential of combining sEV miRNA profiles with existing cancer markers to improve diagnostic precision and sensitivity is particularly promising. Moreover, advancements in sEVs isolation and miRNA detection techniques are crucial for the application of these particles as novel biomarkers in clinical settings. Although the field is still developing, improving in situ detection methods for miRNAs represents a significant step forward. The creation and expansion of comprehensive databases such as ExoCarta, EVpedia, and exRNA Atlas have played a pivotal role in facilitating data sharing and analysis, accelerating research progress in this rapidly evolving field.

Overall, sEVs emanating from the tumour microenvironment possess unique miRNA cargoes that reflect the cellular origins and state of disease progression. The ability to capture these molecular signatures from biofluids and quantify them offers a promising avenue towards the realisation of minimally invasive or non-invasive cancer diagnostics. As we continue to explore the complexities of sEV miRNAs and their interactions within the tumour microenvironment, the prospect of harnessing these entities for the enhancement of cancer diagnosis and the development of personalised medicine approaches becomes increasingly tangible.

Acknowledgements

This work was supported by Apollo Hospitals Educational and Research Foundation (AHERF). We thank our AHERF President, Dr. N.K. Ganguly, Vice president; Ishita Shively, Clinical director; Dr. Jayanthi Swaminathan for active organisational support.

Competing interests

None.

Author details

Sarwareddy Kartik Kumar[1] and Manda Venkata Sasidhar[1,2]*

1 Apollo Hospitals Educational and Research Foundation (AHERF), Apollo Hospitals, Jubilee Hills, Hyderabad, India

2 Urvogelbio Private Limited, AHERF, Jubilee Hills, Hyderabad, India

*Address all correspondence to: sasidhar@aherf.net

References

[1] Chen K, Sun J, Zhao H, Jiang R, Zheng J, Li Z, et al. Non-invasive lung cancer diagnosis and prognosis based on multi-analyte liquid biopsy. Molecular Cancer. 2021;**20**(1):23. Epub 2021/01/31. DOI: 10.1186/s12943-021-01323-9

[2] Braig ZV. Personalized medicine: From diagnostic to adaptive. Biomedical Journal. 2022;**45**(1):132-142. Epub 2022/05/20. DOI: 10.1016/j.bj.2019.05.004

[3] Crosby D, Bhatia S, Brindle KM, Coussens LM, Dive C, Emberton M, et al. Early detection of cancer. Science (New York, NY). 2022;**375**(6586):eaay9040. Epub 2022/03/18. DOI: 10.1126/science.aay9040

[4] Lone SN, Nisar S, Masoodi T, Singh M, Rizwan A, Hashem S, et al. Liquid biopsy: A step closer to transform diagnosis, prognosis and future of cancer treatments. Molecular Cancer. 2022;**21**(1):79. Epub 2022/03/20. DOI: 10.1186/s12943-022-01543-7

[5] Connal S, Cameron JM, Sala A, Brennan PM, Palmer DS, Palmer JD, et al. Liquid biopsies: The future of cancer early detection. Journal of Translational Medicine. 2023;**21**(1):118. Epub 2023/02/12. DOI: 10.1186/s12967-023-03960-8

[6] Kim DH, Kim SW, Hwang SH. Efficacy of non-invasive diagnostic methods in the diagnosis and screening of oral cancer and precancer. Brazilian Journal of Otorhinolaryngology. 2022;**88**(6):937-947. Epub 2021/03/02. DOI: 10.1016/j.bjorl.2020.12.019

[7] Testa A, Venturelli E, Brizzi MF. Extracellular vesicles: New tools for early diagnosis of breast and genitourinary cancers. International Journal of Molecular Sciences. 2021;**22**(16):1-31. Epub 2021/08/28. DOI: 10.3390/ijms22168430

[8] Liu SY, Liao Y, Hosseinifard H, Imani S, Wen QL. Diagnostic role of extracellular vesicles in cancer: A comprehensive systematic review and meta-analysis. Frontiers in Cell and Developmental Biology. 2021;**9**:705791. Epub 2021/11/02. DOI: 10.3389/fcell.2021.705791

[9] Dini L, Tacconi S, Carata E, Tata AM, Vergallo C, Panzarini E. Microvesicles and exosomes in metabolic diseases and inflammation. Cytokine & Growth Factor Reviews. 2020;**51**:27-39. Epub 2020/01/10. DOI: 10.1016/j.cytogfr.2019.12.008

[10] Testa A, Venturelli E, Brizzi MF. Extracellular vesicles as a novel liquid biopsy-based diagnosis for the central nervous system, head and neck, lung, and gastrointestinal cancers: Current and future perspectives. Cancers. 2021;**13**(11):1-30. Epub 2021/07/03. DOI: 10.3390/cancers13112792

[11] Ali Syeda Z, Langden SSS, Munkhzul C, Lee M, Song SJ. Regulatory mechanism of MicroRNA expression in cancer. International Journal of Molecular Sciences. 2020;**21**(5):1-18. Epub 2020/03/07. DOI: 10.3390/ijms21051723

[12] Kciuk M, Yahya EB, Mohamed MMI, Abdulsamad MA, Allaq AA, Gielecińska A, et al. Insights into the role of LncRNAs and miRNAs in glioma progression and their potential as novel therapeutic targets. Cancers.

2023;**15**(13):1-33. Epub 2023/07/14. DOI: 10.3390/cancers15133298

[13] Szczepaniak A, Bronisz A, Godlewski J. Circular RNAs-new kids on the block in cancer pathophysiology and management. Cells. 2023;**12**(4):1-24. Epub 2023/02/26. DOI: 10.3390/cells12040552

[14] Vu LT, Gong J, Pham TT, Kim Y, Le MTN. microRNA exchange via extracellular vesicles in cancer. Cell Proliferation. 2020;**53**(11):e12877. Epub 2020/11/11. DOI: 10.1111/cpr.12877

[15] Bronisz A, Godlewski J, Chiocca EA. Extracellular vesicles and MicroRNAs: Their role in tumorigenicity and therapy for brain tumors. Cellular and Molecular Neurobiology. 2016;**36**(3):361-376. Epub 2016/03/18. DOI: 10.1007/s10571-015-0293-4

[16] Yang Y, Kannisto E, Yu G, Reid ME, Patnaik SK, Wu Y. An immuno-biochip selectively captures tumor-derived exosomes and detects exosomal RNAs for cancer diagnosis. ACS Applied Materials & Interfaces. 2018;**10**(50):43375-43386. Epub 2018/11/20. DOI: 10.1021/acsami.8b13971

[17] Stevic I, Müller V, Weber K, Fasching PA, Karn T, Marmé F, et al. Specific microRNA signatures in exosomes of triple-negative and HER2-positive breast cancer patients undergoing neoadjuvant therapy within the GeparSixto trial. BMC Medicine. 2018;**16**(1):179. Epub 2018/10/12. DOI: 10.1186/s12916-018-1163-y

[18] Wang M, Yu F, Ding H, Wang Y, Li P, Wang K. Emerging function and clinical values of exosomal MicroRNAs in cancer. Molecular Therapy Nucleic Acids. 2019;**16**:791-804. Epub 2019/06/05. DOI: 10.1016/j.omtn.2019.04.027

[19] Dilsiz N. Role of exosomes and exosomal microRNAs in cancer. Future Science OA. 2020;**6**(4):Fso465. Epub 2020/04/08. DOI: 10.2144/fsoa-2019-0116

[20] Juan T, Fürthauer M. Biogenesis and function of ESCRT-dependent extracellular vesicles. Seminars in Cell & Developmental Biology. 2018;**74**:66-77. Epub 2017/08/16. DOI: 10.1016/j.semcdb.2017.08.022

[21] Wollert T, Hurley JH. Molecular mechanism of multivesicular body biogenesis by ESCRT complexes. Nature. 2010;**464**(7290):864-869. Epub 2010/03/23. DOI: 10.1038/nature08849

[22] Yue B, Yang H, Wang J, Ru W, Wu J, Huang Y, et al. Exosome biogenesis, secretion and function of exosomal miRNAs in skeletal muscle myogenesis. Cell Proliferation. 2020;**53**(7):e12857. Epub 2020/06/25. DOI: 10.1111/cpr.12857

[23] Groot M, Lee H. Sorting mechanisms for MicroRNAs into extracellular vesicles and their associated diseases. Cells. 2020;**9**(4):1-16. Epub 2020/04/26. DOI: 10.3390/cells9041044

[24] Lee H, Li C, Zhang Y, Zhang D, Otterbein LE, Jin Y. Caveolin-1 selectively regulates microRNA sorting into microvesicles after noxious stimuli. The Journal of Experimental Medicine. 2019;**216**(9):2202-2220. Epub 2019/06/27. DOI: 10.1084/jem.20182313

[25] Kosaka N, Iguchi H, Yoshioka Y, Takeshita F, Matsuki Y, Ochiya T. Secretory mechanisms and intercellular transfer of microRNAs in living cells. The Journal of Biological Chemistry. 2010;**285**(23):17442-17452. Epub 2010/04/01. DOI: 10.1074/jbc.M110.107821

[26] Wei JX, Lv LH, Wan YL, Cao Y, Li GL, Lin HM, et al. Vps4A functions as a tumor suppressor by regulating the secretion and uptake of exosomal

microRNAs in human hepatoma cells. Hepatology (Baltimore, Md). 2015;**61**(4):1284-1294. Epub 2014/12/17. DOI: 10.1002/hep.27660

[27] Jackson CE, Scruggs BS, Schaffer JE, Hanson PI. Effects of inhibiting VPS4 support a general role for ESCRTs in extracellular vesicle biogenesis. Biophysical Journal. 2017;**113**(6):1342-1352. Epub 2017/06/21. DOI: 10.1016/j.bpj.2017.05.032

[28] Cha DJ, Franklin JL, Dou Y, Liu Q, Higginbotham JN, Demory Beckler M, et al. KRAS-dependent sorting of miRNA to exosomes. eLife. 2015;**4**:e07197. Epub 2015/07/02. DOI: 10.7554/eLife.07197

[29] Melo SA, Sugimoto H, O'Connell JT, Kato N, Villanueva A, Vidal A, et al. Cancer exosomes perform cell-independent microRNA biogenesis and promote tumorigenesis. Cancer Cell. 2014;**26**(5):707-721. Epub 2014/12/03. DOI: 10.1016/j.ccell.2014.09.005

[30] Aseervatham J. Dynamic role of exosome microRNAs in cancer cell signaling and their emerging role as noninvasive biomarkers. Biology. 2023;**12**(5):1-32. Epub 2023/05/27. DOI: 10.3390/biology12050710

[31] Kumar SK, Sasidhar MV. Recent trends in the use of small extracellular vesicles as optimal drug delivery vehicles in oncology. Molecular Pharmaceutics. 2023;**20**(8):3829-3842. Epub 2023/07/06. DOI: 10.1021/acs.molpharmaceut.3c00363

[32] Chen L, Cao P, Huang C, Wu Q, Chen S, Chen F. Serum exosomal miR-7977 as a novel biomarker for lung adenocarcinoma. Journal of Cellular Biochemistry. 2020;**121**(5-6):3382-3391. Epub 2020/01/04. DOI: 10.1002/jcb.29612

[33] Feng M, Zhao J, Wang L, Liu J. Upregulated expression of serum exosomal microRNAs as diagnostic biomarkers of lung adenocarcinoma. Annals of Clinical and Laboratory Science. 2018;**48**(6):712-718. Epub 2019/01/06

[34] Wu Q, Yu L, Lin X, Zheng Q, Zhang S, Chen D, et al. Combination of serum miRNAs with serum exosomal miRNAs in early diagnosis for non-small-cell lung cancer. Cancer Management and Research. 2020;**12**:485-495. Epub 2020/02/06. DOI: 10.2147/cmar.S232383

[35] Tang Y, Zhang Z, Song X, Yu M, Niu L, Zhao Y, et al. Tumor-derived exosomal miR-620 as a diagnostic biomarker in non-small-cell lung cancer. Journal of Oncology. 2020;**2020**:6691211. Epub 2020/12/22. DOI: 10.1155/2020/6691211

[36] Zhang ZJ, Song XG, Xie L, Wang KY, Tang YY, Yu M, et al. Circulating serum exosomal miR-20b-5p and miR-3187-5p as efficient diagnostic biomarkers for early-stage non-small cell lung cancer. Experimental Biology and Medicine (Maywood, NJ). 2020;**245**(16):1428-1436. Epub 2020/08/04. DOI: 10.1177/1535370220945987

[37] Zhang Y, Zhang Y, Yin Y, Li S. Detection of circulating exosomal miR-17-5p serves as a novel non-invasive diagnostic marker for non-small cell lung cancer patients. Pathology, Research and Practice. 2019;**215**(8):152466. Epub 2019/05/31. DOI: 10.1016/j.prp.2019.152466

[38] Yang G, Wang T, Qu X, Chen S, Han Z, Chen S, et al. Exosomal miR-21/Let-7a ratio distinguishes non-small cell lung cancer from benign pulmonary diseases. Asia-Pacific Journal of Clinical Oncology. 2020;**16**(4):280-286. Epub 2020/06/12. DOI: 10.1111/ajco.13343

[39] Kanaoka R, Iinuma H, Dejima H, Sakai T, Uehara H, Matsutani N,

et al. Usefulness of plasma exosomal MicroRNA-451a as a noninvasive biomarker for early prediction of recurrence and prognosis of non-small cell lung cancer. Oncology. 2018;**94**(5):311-323. Epub 2018/03/14. DOI: 10.1159/000487006

[40] Grimolizzi F, Monaco F, Leoni F, Bracci M, Staffolani S, Bersaglieri C, et al. Exosomal miR-126 as a circulating biomarker in non-small-cell lung cancer regulating cancer progression. Scientific Reports. 2017;**7**(1):15277. Epub 2017/11/12. DOI: 10.1038/s41598-017-15475-6

[41] Eichelser C, Stückrath I, Müller V, Milde-Langosch K, Wikman H, Pantel K, et al. Increased serum levels of circulating exosomal microRNA-373 in receptor-negative breast cancer patients. Oncotarget. 2014;**5**(20):9650-9663. Epub 2014/10/22. DOI: 10.18632/oncotarget.2520

[42] Zhai LY, Li MX, Pan WL, Chen Y, Li MM, Pang JX, et al. In situ detection of plasma exosomal MicroRNA-1246 for breast cancer diagnostics by a Au nanoflare probe. ACS Applied Materials & Interfaces. 2018;**10**(46):39478-39486. Epub 2018/10/24. DOI: 10.1021/acsami.8b12725

[43] Yoshikawa M, Iinuma H, Umemoto Y, Yanagisawa T, Matsumoto A, Jinno H. Exosome-encapsulated microRNA-223-3p as a minimally invasive biomarker for the early detection of invasive breast cancer. Oncology Letters. 2018;**15**(6):9584-9592. Epub 2018/05/29. DOI: 10.3892/ol.2018.8457

[44] Asadirad A, Khodadadi A, Talaiezadeh A, Shohan M, Rashno M, Joudaki N. Evaluation of miRNA-21-5p and miRNA-10b-5p levels in serum-derived exosomes of breast cancer patients in different grades. Molecular and Cellular Probes. 2022;**64**:101831. Epub 2022/06/07. DOI: 10.1016/j.mcp.2022.101831

[45] Qin X, Xiang Y, Li N, Wei B, Chen Y, Fang D, et al. Simultaneous detection of cancerous exosomal miRNA-21 and PD-L1 with a sensitive dual-cycling nanoprobe. Biosensors & Bioelectronics. 2022;**216**:114636. Epub 2022/08/21. DOI: 10.1016/j.bios.2022.114636

[46] Shi R, Wang PY, Li XY, Chen JX, Li Y, Zhang XZ, et al. Exosomal levels of miRNA-21 from cerebrospinal fluids associated with poor prognosis and tumor recurrence of glioma patients. Oncotarget. 2015;**6**(29):26971-26981. Epub 2015/08/19. DOI: 10.18632/oncotarget.4699

[47] Lan F, Qing Q, Pan Q, Hu M, Yu H, Yue X. Serum exosomal miR-301a as a potential diagnostic and prognostic biomarker for human glioma. Cellular Oncology (Dordrecht). 2018;**41**(1):25-33. Epub 2017/10/28. DOI: 10.1007/s13402-017-0355-3

[48] Lan F, Yue X, Xia T. Exosomal microRNA-210 is a potentially non-invasive biomarker for the diagnosis and prognosis of glioma. Oncology Letters. 2020;**19**(3):1967-1974. Epub 2020/03/21. DOI: 10.3892/ol.2020.11249

[49] Sun J, Sun Z, Gareev I, Yan T, Chen X, Ahmad A, et al. Exosomal miR-2276-5p in plasma is a potential diagnostic and prognostic biomarker in glioma. Frontiers in Cell and Developmental Biology. 2021;**9**:671202. Epub 2021/06/19. DOI: 10.3389/fcell.2021.671202

[50] Liu W, Yang D, Chen L, Liu Q, Wang W, Yang Z, et al. Plasma exosomal miRNA-139-3p is a novel biomarker of colorectal cancer. Journal of Cancer. 2020;**11**(16):4899-4906. Epub 2020/07/07. DOI: 10.7150/jca.45548

[51] Wang L, Song X, Yu M, Niu L, Zhao Y, Tang Y, et al. Serum exosomal miR-377-3p and miR-381-3p as diagnostic biomarkers in colorectal cancer. Future Oncology (London, England). 2022;**18**(7):793-805. Epub 2021/12/03. DOI: 10.2217/fon-2021-1130

[52] Wu J, Lin B, Yu S, Chen Y, Chen J, Li C, et al. Exosomal miR-196b-5p is a potential diagnostic marker for colorectal cancer with metachronous liver metastasis. Translational Cancer Research. 2018;**7**(6):1482-1490

[53] Li Z, Ma YY, Wang J, Zeng XF, Li R, Kang W, et al. Exosomal microRNA-141 is upregulated in the serum of prostate cancer patients. OncoTargets and Therapy. 2016;**9**:139-148. Epub 2016/01/16. DOI: 10.2147/ott.S95565

[54] Matsuzaki K, Fujita K, Tomiyama E, Hatano K, Hayashi Y, Wang C, et al. MiR-30b-3p and miR-126-3p of urinary extracellular vesicles could be new biomarkers for prostate cancer. Translational Andrology and Urology. 2021;**10**(4):1918-1927. Epub 2021/05/11. DOI: 10.21037/tau-20-421

[55] Zhai TY, Dou M, Ma YB, Wang H, Liu F, Zhang LD, et al. miR-20b-5p is a novel biomarker for detecting prostate cancer. Oncology Letters. 2022;**24**(6):426. Epub 2022/11/01. DOI: 10.3892/ol.2022.13546

[56] Wang Y, Fang YX, Dong B, Du X, Wang J, Wang X, et al. Discovery of extracellular vesicles derived miR-181a-5p in patient's serum as an indicator for bone-metastatic prostate cancer. Theranostics. 2021;**11**(2):878-892. Epub 2021/01/05. DOI: 10.7150/thno.49186

[57] Yokoi A, Yoshioka Y, Hirakawa A, Yamamoto Y, Ishikawa M, Ikeda SI, et al. A combination of circulating miRNAs for the early detection of ovarian cancer. Oncotarget. 2017;**8**(52):89811-89823. Epub 2017/11/23. DOI: 10.18632/oncotarget.20688

[58] Kim S, Choi MC, Jeong JY, Hwang S, Jung SG, Joo WD, et al. Serum exosomal miRNA-145 and miRNA-200c as promising biomarkers for preoperative diagnosis of ovarian carcinomas. Journal of Cancer. 2019;**10**(9):1958-1967. Epub 2019/06/18. DOI: 10.7150/jca.30231

[59] Soeda N, Iinuma H, Suzuki Y, Tsukahara D, Midorikawa H, Igarashi Y, et al. Plasma exosome-encapsulated microRNA-21 and microRNA-92a are promising biomarkers for the prediction of peritoneal recurrence in patients with gastric cancer. Oncology Letters. 2019;**18**(5):4467-4480. Epub 2019/10/16. DOI: 10.3892/ol.2019.10807

[60] Cho HJ, Baek GO, Seo CW, Ahn HR, Sung S, Son JA, et al. Exosomal microRNA-4661-5p-based serum panel as a potential diagnostic biomarker for early-stage hepatocellular carcinoma. Cancer Medicine. 2020;**9**(15):5459-5472. Epub 2020/06/17. DOI: 10.1002/cam4.3230

[61] Wang H, Hou L, Li A, Duan Y, Gao H, Song X. Expression of serum exosomal microRNA-21 in human hepatocellular carcinoma. BioMed Research International. 2014;**2014**:864894. Epub 2014/06/26. DOI: 10.1155/2014/864894

[62] Wen Q, Wang Y, Li X, Jin X, Wang G. Decreased serum exosomal miR-29a expression and its clinical significance in papillary thyroid carcinoma. Journal of Clinical Laboratory Analysis. 2021;**35**(1):e23560. Epub 2020/12/29. DOI: 10.1002/jcla.23560

[63] El-Shal AS, Shalaby SM, Abouhashem SE, Elbary EHA, Azazy S,

Rashad NM, et al. Urinary exosomal microRNA-96-5p and microRNA-183-5p expression as potential biomarkers of bladder cancer. Molecular Biology Reports. 2021;**48**(5):4361-4371. Epub 2021/06/05. DOI: 10.1007/s11033-021-06451-5

[64] He T, Guo X, Li X, Liao C, Wang X, He K. Plasma-derived exosomal microRNA-130a serves as a noninvasive biomarker for diagnosis and prognosis of oral squamous cell carcinoma. Journal of Oncology. 2021;**2021**:5547911. DOI: 10.1155/2021/5547911

[65] Wang C, Ding Q, Plant P, Basheer M, Yang C, Tawedrous E, et al. Droplet digital PCR improves urinary exosomal miRNA detection compared to real-time PCR. Clinical Biochemistry. 2019;**67**:54-59. Epub 2019/03/25. DOI: 10.1016/j.clinbiochem.2019.03.008

[66] Luo L, Wang L, Zeng L, Wang Y, Weng Y, Liao Y, et al. A ratiometric electrochemical DNA biosensor for detection of exosomal MicroRNA. Talanta. 2020;**207**:120298. Epub 2019/10/09. DOI: 10.1016/j.talanta.2019.120298

[67] Li X, Li X, Li D, Zhao M, Wu H, Shen B, et al. Electrochemical biosensor for ultrasensitive exosomal miRNA analysis by cascade primer exchange reaction and MOF@Pt@MOF nanozyme. Biosensors & Bioelectronics. 2020;**168**:112554. Epub 2020/09/02. DOI: 10.1016/j.bios.2020.112554

[68] Zhao Y, Fang X, Bai M, Zhang J, Yu H, Chen F, et al. A microfluidic surface-enhanced Raman scattering (SERS) sensor for microRNA in extracellular vesicles with nucleic acid-tyramine cascade amplification. Chinese Chemical Letters. 2022;**33**(4):2101-2104. DOI: 10.1016/j.cclet.2021.08.047

[69] Xia Y, Chen T, Zhang L, Zhang X, Shi W, Chen G, et al. Colorimetric detection of exosomal microRNA through switching the visible-light-induced oxidase mimic activity of acridone derivate. Biosensors and Bioelectronics. 2021;**173**:112834. DOI: 10.1016/j.bios.2020.112834

[70] Yasui T, Yanagida T, Ito S, Konakade Y, Takeshita D, Naganawa T, et al. Unveiling massive numbers of cancer-related urinary-microRNA candidates via nanowires. Science Advances. 2017;**3**(12):e1701133. Epub 2018/01/02. DOI: 10.1126/sciadv.1701133

[71] Zhang XW, Du L, Liu MX, Wang JH, Chen S, Yu YL. All-in-one nanoflare biosensor combined with catalyzed hairpin assembly amplification for in situ and sensitive exosomal miRNA detection and cancer classification. Talanta. 2024;**266**(Pt 2):125145. Epub 2023/09/04. DOI: 10.1016/j.talanta.2023.125145

[72] Zhou X, Tang W, Zhang Y, Deng A, Guo Y, Qian L. Liposome-exosome hybrids for in situ detection of exosomal miR-1246 in breast cancer. The Analyst. 2024;**149**(2):403-409. Epub 2023/12/07. DOI: 10.1039/d3an01600e

[73] Rabinowits G, Gerçel-Taylor C, Day JM, Taylor DD, Kloecker GH. Exosomal microRNA: A diagnostic marker for lung cancer. Clinical Lung Cancer. 2009;**10**(1):42-46. Epub 2009/03/18. DOI: 10.3816/CLC.2009.n.006

[74] Nilsson J, Skog J, Nordstrand A, Baranov V, Mincheva-Nilsson L, Breakefield XO, et al. Prostate cancer-derived urine exosomes: A novel approach to biomarkers for prostate cancer. British Journal of Cancer. 2009;**100**(10):1603-1607. Epub 2009/04/30. DOI: 10.1038/sj.bjc.6605058

[75] Ohshima K, Inoue K, Fujiwara A, Hatakeyama K, Kanto K, Watanabe Y, et al. Let-7 microRNA family is selectively secreted into the extracellular environment via exosomes in a metastatic gastric cancer cell line. PLoS One. 2010;**5**(10):e13247. Epub 2010/10/16. DOI: 10.1371/journal.pone.0013247

[76] Hong F, Li N, Feng Z, Zheng Y, Zhu C, Zhang F. Exosomal microRNAs as novel diagnostic biomarkers in breast cancer: A systematic evaluation and meta-analysis. Asian Journal of Surgery. 2023;**46**(11):4727-4736. DOI: 10.1016/j.asjsur.2023.05.115

[77] Chen Y, Zhai LY, Zhang LM, Ma XS, Liu Z, Li MM, et al. Breast cancer plasma biopsy by in situ determination of exosomal microRNA-1246 with a molecular beacon. The Analyst. 2021;**146**(7):2264-2276. Epub 2021/02/19. DOI: 10.1039/d0an02224a

[78] Tang Y, Zhao Y, Song X, Song X, Niu L, Xie L. Tumor-derived exosomal miRNA-320d as a biomarker for metastatic colorectal cancer. Journal of Clinical Laboratory Analysis. 2019;**33**(9):e23004. Epub 2019/08/20. DOI: 10.1002/jcla.23004

[79] Wang J, Yan F, Zhao Q, Zhan F, Wang R, Wang L, et al. Circulating exosomal miR-125a-3p as a novel biomarker for early-stage colon cancer. Scientific Reports. 2017;**7**(1):4150. Epub 2017/06/25. DOI: 10.1038/s41598-017-04386-1

[80] Sun L, Liu X, Pan B, Hu X, Zhu Y, Su Y, et al. Serum exosomal miR-122 as a potential diagnostic and prognostic biomarker of colorectal cancer with liver metastasis. Journal of Cancer. 2020;**11**(3):630-637. Epub 2020/01/17. DOI: 10.7150/jca.33022

[81] Han J, Sun W, Liu R, Zhou Z, Zhang H, Chen X, et al. Plasma exosomal miRNA expression profile as oxaliplatin-based chemoresistant biomarkers in colorectal adenocarcinoma. Frontiers in Oncology. 2020;**10**:1495. Epub 2020/10/20. DOI: 10.3389/fonc.2020.01495

[82] Ma J, Wang P, Huang L, Qiao J, Li J. Bioinformatic analysis reveals an exosomal miRNA-mRNA network in colorectal cancer. BMC Medical Genomics. 2021;**14**(1):60. Epub 2021/03/01. DOI: 10.1186/s12920-021-00905-2

[83] Ramirez-Garrastacho M, Berge V, Linē A, Llorente A. Potential of miRNAs in urinary extracellular vesicles for management of active surveillance in prostate cancer patients. British Journal of Cancer. 2022;**126**(3):492-501. Epub 2021/11/24. DOI: 10.1038/s41416-021-01598-1

[84] Lu Z, Hou J, Li X, Zhou J, Luo B, Liang S, et al. Exosome-derived miRNAs as potential biomarkers for prostate bone metastasis. International Journal of General Medicine. 2022;**15**:5369-5383. Epub 2022/06/09. DOI: 10.2147/ijgm.S361981

[85] Lin H, Shi X, Li H, Hui J, Liu R, Chen Z, et al. Urinary exosomal miRNAs as biomarkers of bladder cancer and experimental verification of mechanism of miR-93-5p in bladder cancer. BMC Cancer. 2021;**21**(1):1293. Epub 2021/12/05. DOI: 10.1186/s12885-021-08926-x

[86] Kumata Y, Iinuma H, Suzuki Y, Tsukahara D, Midorikawa H, Igarashi Y, et al. Exosome-encapsulated microRNA-23b as a minimally invasive liquid biomarker for the prediction of recurrence and prognosis of gastric cancer patients in each tumor stage. Oncology Reports. 2018;**40**(1):319-330. Epub 2018/05/12. DOI: 10.3892/or.2018.6418

[87] Wang Y, Zhang C, Zhang P, Guo G, Jiang T, Zhao X, et al. Serum exosomal microRNAs combined with alpha-fetoprotein as diagnostic markers of hepatocellular carcinoma. Cancer Medicine. 2018;**7**(5):1670-1679. Epub 2018/03/25. DOI: 10.1002/cam4.1390

[88] Chen S, Mao Y, Chen W, Liu C, Wu H, Zhang J, et al. Serum exosomal miR-34a as a potential biomarker for the diagnosis and prognostic of hepatocellular carcinoma. Journal of Cancer. 2022;**13**(5):1410-1417. Epub 2022/04/05. DOI: 10.7150/jca.57205

[89] Jiang K, Li G, Chen W, Song L, Wei T, Li Z, et al. Plasma exosomal miR-146b-5p and miR-222-3p are potential biomarkers for lymph node metastasis in papillary thyroid carcinomas. OncoTargets and Therapy. 2020;**13**:1311-1319. Epub 2020/02/28. DOI: 10.2147/ott.S231361

[90] Faur CI, Roman RC, Jurj A, Raduly L, Almăşan O, Rotaru H, et al. Salivary exosomal MicroRNA-486-5p and MicroRNA-10b-5p in oral and oropharyngeal squamous cell carcinoma. Medicina (Kaunas, Lithuania). 2022;**58**(10). Epub 2022/10/28. DOI: 10.3390/medicina58101478

[91] Keerthikumar S, Chisanga D, Ariyaratne D, Al Saffar H, Anand S, Zhao K, et al. ExoCarta: A web-based compendium of exosomal cargo. Journal of Molecular Biology. 2016;**428**(4):688-692. DOI: 10.1016/j.jmb.2015.09.019

[92] Mathivanan S, Fahner CJ, Reid GE, Simpson RJ. ExoCarta 2012: Database of exosomal proteins. RNA and Lipids. Nucleic Acids Research. 2011;**40**(D1):D1241-D12D4. DOI: 10.1093/nar/gkr828 %J Nucleic Acids Research

[93] Kim DK, Kang B, Kim OY, Choi DS, Lee J, Kim SR, et al. EVpedia: An integrated database of high-throughput data for systemic analyses of extracellular vesicles. Journal of Extracellular Vesicles. 2013;**2**:1-7. Epub 2013/09/07. DOI: 10.3402/jev.v2i0.20384

[94] Chitti SV, Gummadi S, Kang T, Shahi S, Marzan AL, Nedeva C, et al. Vesiclepedia 2024: An extracellular vesicles and extracellular particles repository. Nucleic Acids Research. 2024;**52**(D1):D1694-D16d8. Epub 2023/11/13. DOI: 10.1093/nar/gkad1007

[95] Murillo OD, Thistlethwaite W, Rozowsky J, Subramanian SL, Lucero R, Shah N, et al. exRNA atlas analysis reveals distinct extracellular RNA cargo types and their carriers present across human biofluids. Cell. 2019;**177**(2):463-77.e15. Epub 2019/04/06. DOI: 10.1016/j.cell.2019.02.018

[96] Lai H, Li Y, Zhang H, Hu J, Liao J, Su Y, et al. exoRBase 2.0: An atlas of mRNA, lncRNA and circRNA in extracellular vesicles from human biofluids. Nucleic Acids Research. 2022;**50**(D1):D118-Dd28. Epub 2021/12/18. DOI: 10.1093/nar/gkab1085

[97] Russo F, Di Bella S, Nigita G, Macca V, Laganà A, Giugno R, et al. miRandola: extracellular circulating microRNAs database. PloS One. 2012;**7**(10):e47786. Epub 2012/10/25. DOI: 10.1371/journal.pone.0047786

Chapter 4

Gene Regulation via RNA Isoform Variations

Bin Zhang and Chenchеng Xu

Abstract

The completion of the draft and complete human genome has revealed that there are only around 20,000 genes encoding proteins. Nonetheless, these genes can generate eight times more RNA transcript isoforms, while this number is still growing with the accumulation of high-throughput RNA sequencing (RNA-seq) data. In general, over 90% of genes generate various RNA isoforms emerging from variations at the 5′ and 3′ ends, as well as different exon combinations, known as alternative transcription start site (TSS), alternative polyadenylation (APA), and alternative splicing (AS). In this chapter, our focus will be on introducing the significance of these three types of isoform variations in gene regulation and their underlying molecular mechanisms. Additionally, we will highlight the historical, current, and prospective technological advancements in elucidating isoform regulations, from both the computational side such as deep-learning-based artificial intelligence, and the experimental aspect such as the long-read third-generation sequencing (TGS).

Keywords: gene regulation, RNA isoform, RNA-seq, next generation sequencing, third generation sequencing, transcription start site, alternative splicing, alternative polyadenylation, deep learning

1. Introduction

Since the initial release of the human genome draft in 2001 [1, 2], gaps or unplaced sequences in the genome have been solved continuously. In 2022, the telomere-to-telomere (T2T) consortium published the first complete sequence of a human genome [3]. With these genome sequences as the reference, genes have been annotated accordingly and now it is well accepted that there are only around 20,000 genes encoding proteins in the human genome. For instance, based on the GENCODE annotation database [4], the number of protein-coding gene (PCG) has been almost invariable in the last decade (**Figure 1A**). However, the number of annotated RNA transcripts transcribed from these genes gradually increased (**Figure 1B**). In general, over 90% of them transcribed multiple RNA transcripts known as isoforms, with variations at 5′ and 3′ end, as well as different exon combinations (**Figure 1C**).

The variation at the 5′ and 3′ end of isoforms are known as alternative transcription start site (TSS) and alternative polyadenylation (APA), respectively, whereas isoform variations formed by different exon combinations are mediated by alternative splicing (AS). The three types of variations occur at different stages of RNA

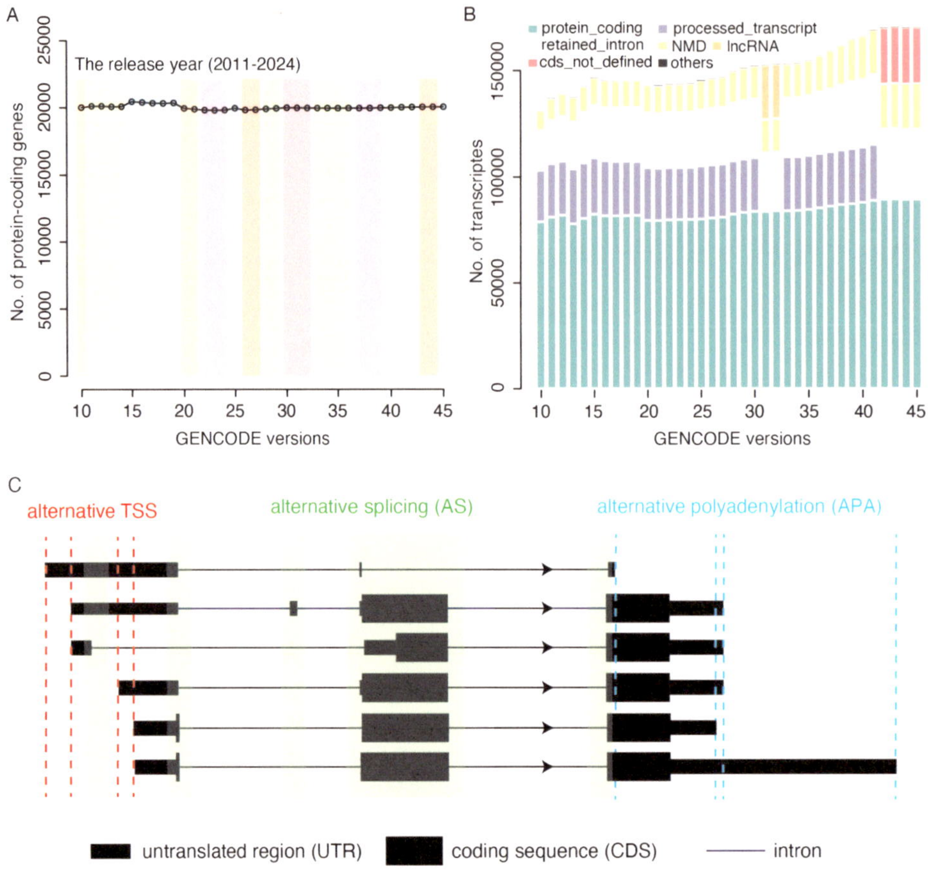

Figure 1.
The number of annotated genes encoding a protein (A) and transcripts transcribed from these genes (B) in the GENCODE database since 2011. The X-axis in (A) and (B) is the released versions of GENCODE annotations. Each dot in (A) represents the number of genes in each release and the segmented colors indicate the released years. Bars in (B) are colored for different transcript types, in which NMD stands for nonsense mediated decay. In general, transcripts transcribed from PCGs are classified into four types, including protein_coding, process_transcript, retained_intron, and NMD. The classification is based on their coding potential (protein_coding) and other properties, such as whether containing un-spliced introns (retained_intron) or premature termination codons that trigger mRNA degradation (NMD). To be noted, the GENCODE transcript type 'processed_transcript' was defined as long noncoding RNA ('lncRNA') in v31 and v32, and has been redefined as 'protein_coding_CDS_not_defined' since v42.

processing. TSS selection happens when transcription is initiated, and RNA splicing is a posttranscriptional or co-transcriptional process [5]. During transcription termination, nascent RNA molecules undergo cleavage and the addition of poly-adenosine (poly-A) tails, known as polyadenylation [6]. APA involves utilizing varied polyadenylation sites (PASs) to generate isoforms with distinct 3′ ends. In Section 2, we will introduce the molecular mechanisms underlying these three types of variations.

The variable RNA isoforms not only enable the limited number of genes to generate a much larger number of proteins but also greatly increase the complexity of gene regulation even when variations only impact the noncoding sequences of RNA. Dysregulated isoform variations contribute significantly to pathogenesis as they impair the tightly controlled gene regulations. For instance, approximately 15–50% of human genetic disorders are caused by mutations impairing RNA splicing [7].

In cancer, mutations impairing splicing are also frequent, resulting in widespread dysregulated splicing events. Besides, cancer cells expressed isoforms utilizing distinct PAS. In addition, pervasive regulations of TSS through alternative promoters have been observed in tumor samples [8]. These dysregulations cover both coding sequence (CDS) and noncoding sequence of RNA, such as untranslated region (UTR) and intron. The detailed functional consequence of isoform variations at the molecular and cellular level will be elucidated in Section 3 and their dysregulations in human disease will be introduced in Section 4.

In the last two decades, the next generation sequencing (NGS), has revolutionized RNA profiling for different cell types or cells under different conditions [9]. While the primary goal of the profiling is to quantify expression at the gene level, there are still many endeavors focusing on isoform variations, mainly for alternative splicing since its quantification is easier than that of TSS and APA. Hence, specialized experimental protocols have been designed to more effectively capture TSS or PAS. Computational methods have also been developed for detecting them from conventional RNA sequencing (RNA-seq) data despite the performances remaining far from satisfactory.

In the last section of this chapter, we will list the impactive experimental and computational methods for identifying and quantifying the three types of isoform variations. In addition, with the technological advancements of machine learning, enormous methods and models have been proposed for predicting alternative TSS, splicing, and polyadenylation using DNA/RNA sequences as inputs. Their performance continuously improved and many tools become promising for evaluating impact of genetic variants in isoform variations and further predicting the disease risks. However, all these methods are limited to variations at the event level, and overlook the full-length sequence of isoforms. Consequently, at the end of this chapter, we will highlight the powerfulness of third-generation sequencing (TGS) in detecting full-length isoform variations and its potential for training the nature of intact RNA molecule-centric deep-learning models.

2. Molecular mechanisms underlying RNA isoform variations

Gene regulation usually relies on the binding or recruitment of trans-acting factors on cis- elements resigning in DNA or RNA. The regulation of TSS, polyadenylation, and splicing will be introduced separately. At the end of this section, we will highlight the links among these three types of regulations.

2.1 TSS regulation

TSS is determined by the assembly of a transcriptional initiation complex comprising transcriptional machinery such as RNA polymerase and general transcription factors (GTFs) at core promoters [10]. Promoters share various common sequence features, as the most well-documented motif is the TATA-box (TATAWAW) first identified in 1978 [11]. Furthermore, the assembly process is regulated by transcription factors (TFs) and their cofactors that bind to enhancers. Recent studies revealed that these factors form condensates, a liquid-phase-like membrane-less organelle, to coordinate transcription initiation and elongation [12]. Different TFs have distinct sequence binding preferences in DNA, thereby shaping the varied landscape of activated promoters across different cell types and tissues. In addition, whether to utilize a promoter for transcribing RNA is also controlled by epigenetic information, such as nucleosome-free positions, DNA methylation, and posttranslational modifications on histones. Overall, the availability of different TFs and heterogenous promoter epigenetic modifications together regulates alternative TSS utilization (**Figure 2A**).

2.2 Polyadenylation and alternative polyadenylation (APA)

On the other hand, polyadenylation is mainly regulated by several groups of RNA-binding proteins (RBPs), including cleavage and polyadenylation specificity factors (CPSF), cleavage stimulation factors (CstF), and so on (**Figure 2B**). During transcription termination, RNA polymerase pauses downstream of the cleavage/polyadenylation site (PAS), thereafter CPSF and CstF complex are recruited *via* recognizing motifs on the nascent RNA [6]. The hexamer sequence AAUAAA, also called PAS signal or PAS motif, located 15–40 nt upstream of the cleavage site, is the most important cis-element for polyadenylation [13]. Overall, within 50 nt sequences

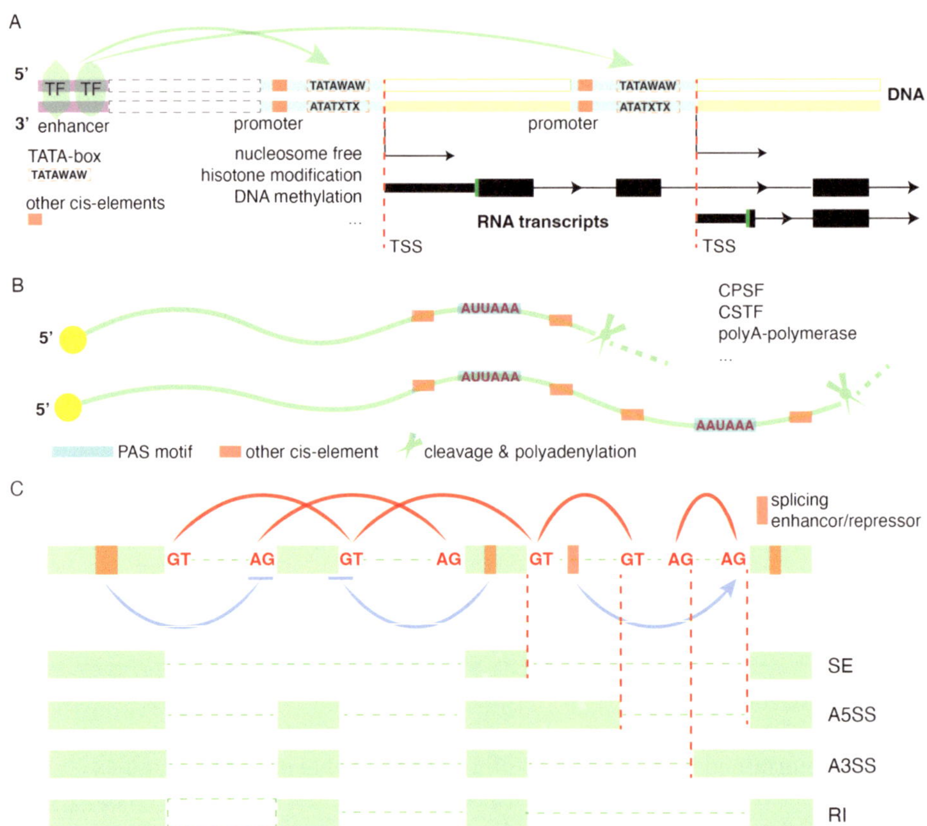

Figure 2.
The schematics show the regulation of alternative TSS (A), polyadenylation (B), and splicing (C). (A) TSS is determined by the core promoter, whose activation depends on the binding of transcription factors (TFs) at the upstream enhancer regions, epigenetic markers, and nucleosome positions. (B) Polyadenylation is regulated by a protein complex, including cleavage and polyadenylation specificity factors (CPSF), cleavage stimulation factors (CSTF), polyA polymerase, and so on. (C) The regulation of alternative splicing is very complicated, for which different splice sites can compete with each other. Moreover, elements within exonic and intronic regions could also enhance (splicing enhancer) or repress (splicing repressor) the splicing. The complex regulations result in multiple types of alternative splicing events, such as skipped exon (SE), alternative 5′ and 3′ splice site (A5SS and A3SS), and retained intron (RI).

upstream of polyadenylation sites (PASs) in human and mouse genomes, more than half of them contain AATAAA and 80% of the rest harbors its variants such as ATTAAA [14, 15]. Alternative utilization of PAS (APA) is regulated by trans-factors enhancing or inhibiting polyadenylation. For instance, RNA binding protein (RBP) NUDT21 (also known as CFIm25) can repress proximal PAS usage in 3′ UTR, and its downregulation results in 3′ UTR shortening in glioblastoma [16].

2.3 Splicing and alternative splicing

Nevertheless, splicing regulation is even more sophisticated, in which spliceosome, the largest protein complex in human cells that also consists of small nuclear RNAs (snRNA), recognizes donor and acceptor splice sites (SSs) in RNA to define exons [17]. The core component of spliceosome is small nuclear ribonucleoproteins (snRNPs) consisting of snRNA and Sm protein or like Sm (LSm) proteins. The U1, U2, U4, U5, and U6 snRNPs regulate >99% of splicing events, while their variant, so-called minor spliceosome formed by the U11, U12, U4atac and U6atac, and U5 regulate the rest of splicing events [18, 19]. snRNPs difference of the two spliceosomes result in two types of introns. The major ones or U2-types start with almost invariable GU dinucleotides at the 5′ splice site (SS) and end with AG dinucleotides at the 3′ SS, whereas U12-type introns start with GU or AU and end with AC or AG [20]. Classically, the 9 nt sequence (−3 to +6) around 5′ SS, and the 23 nt sequence (−20 to +3) around 3′ SS are used for calculating splicing strength, respectively [21].

During RNA maturation, introns are removed, and the two flanking exons are joined together. However, multiple SSs from the same gene can compete with each other, resulting in variable exon definitions and leading to complicated forms of alternative splicing, such as skipping single or multiple exons (SE), retaining introns (RI), and utilizing non-canonical 5′ SS or 3′ SS (A5SS and A3SS) (**Figure 2C**). Even more surprisingly, studies revealed that downstream exons can be back-spliced to join upstream exons, which generates RNA circles or so-called circular RNA [22–24]. In addition to the core spliceosome, other trans-factors also contribute to splicing *via* enhancing or repressing the definition of exons through the interaction with the core spliceosome, further increasing the complexity of splicing choice. Overall, the largest proportion of human isoform variations are from alternative splicing.

2.4 Crosstalk among the three types of variations

Despite the distinct molecular mechanisms underlying alternative TSS, polyadenylation, and splicing, the regulation of these variations is not fully independent. Intuitively, utilizing alternative TSS is associated with alternative splicing of the first exon, while alternative splicing of the last exon impacts the choice of polyadenylation site. In addition, the PAS signal is present in almost every intron in the human genome, suggesting a balance between removing intron by splicing or termination of transcription by polyadenylation. Indeed, studies reveal that U1 snRNP protects pre-mRNA from drastic pre-mature termination at PAS in introns [25], and U1 motifs and PAS signals together shape the landscape of promoter directions [26]. Interestingly, a recent study reveals that the choice of 3′ ends for polyadenylation is globally influenced by the selection of TSS [27], suggesting couplings among the regulation for three types of variations.

3. Functional consequence of RNA isoform variations

In general, isoform variations have three kinds of consequences, including (a) altering open reading frame (ORF) including truncation, (b) changing noncoding sequence of RNA such as untranslated regions (UTR), and (c) triggering mRNA degradation *via* introducing pre-mature termination codon (PTC) or frameshift. Alternative TSS can impact 5′ untranslated region (5′ UTR) or alter N-terminal or even the complete ORF (**Figure 3A**). Similarly, APA can regulate the shortening or lengthening of 3′ UTRs and change C-terminal of the ORF (**Figure 3B**). Traditionally, splicing has been investigated predominantly in coding sequence (CDS), which either leads to ORF alterations or message RNA (mRNA) degradation *via* introducing PTC. However, our recent study reveals pervasive splicing within 3′ UTR [28], indicating AS influences cover all three kinds of consequences (**Figure 3C**).

While ORF alterations can drastically impact functions of the encoded protein, noncoding sequences changes mainly regulate the final protein production. For instance, varied 5′ UTR affect mRNA translation efficiency [29], while 3′ UTR variations regulate mRNA stability and translation efficiency [30]. mRNA degradation *via* introducing PTC usually results in loss of function and its eventual effect depends

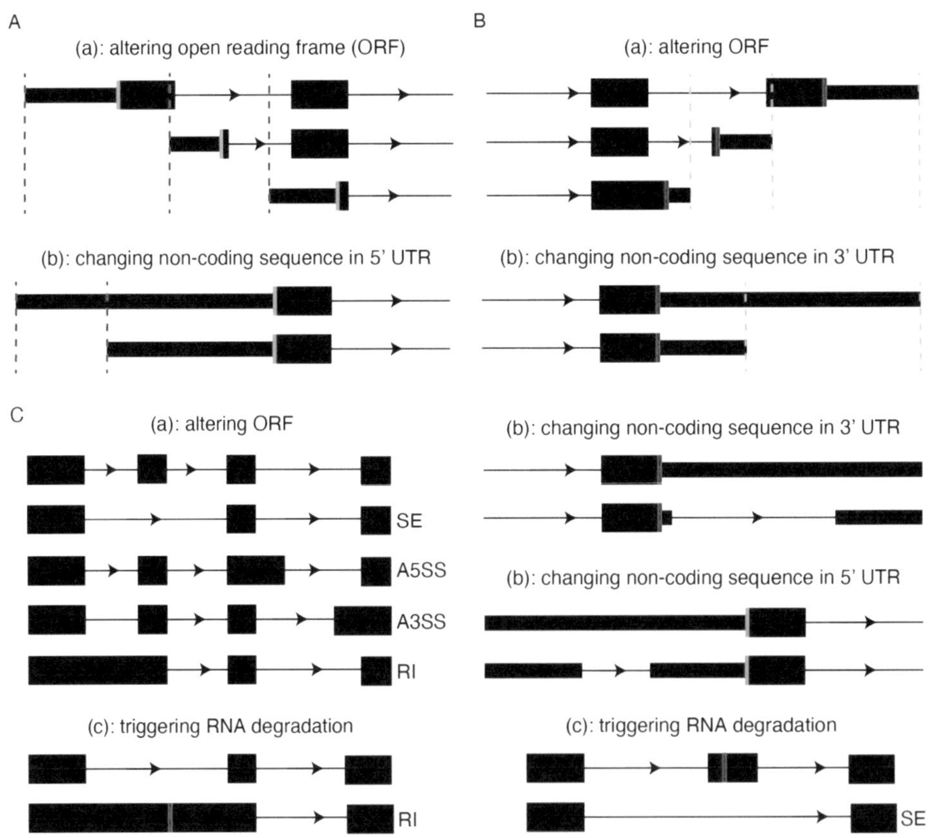

Figure 3.
Three kinds of consequences induced by alternative TSS (A), polyadenylation (B), and splicing (C) at the molecular level. SE: skipped exon; A5SS and A3SS: alternative 5′ and 3′ splice site; RI: retained intron. The narrow green and red bars indicate the start and end codon, respectively.

on the proportion of the isoform. For instance, widespread intron retention has a moderate effect on gene regulation by tuning mammalian tissue RNA expression [31]. Besides, conserved cassette exons containing PTC in the brain are particularly enriched in RBPs, such as splicing factors and other RNA metabolic process regulators, which enables potential gene autoregulation [32].

3.1 Isoform variations regulate biological processes at the cellular level

Since isoform variations or switches have broad impacts on gene expression, they induce diverse functional consequences at the cellular level. An interesting example is about cell stemness and differentiation, where splicing has been the most extensively investigated. For instance, a conserved AS event controls the inclusion or exclusion of a cassette exon in FOXP1 that encodes the protein domain for DNA binding preference, further regulating embryonic stem cell pluripotency and reprogramming [33]. Besides, intron retention changes in a group of genes, including Lmnb1, regulate granulocyte differentiation *via* degradation of intron-retained RNA isoforms by nonsense mediated decay (NMD) [34].

In addition to AS, APA also contributes significantly to cell fate commitment, as evident by the perturbation of NUDT21, an APA regulator controlling 3′ UTR lengthening or shortening for thousands of transcripts [35]. Beyond differentiation, AS and APA are both capable of regulating cell proliferation and cell cycle progression. An interesting phenomenon is that active proliferated cells tend to express isoform with shortened 3′ UTR *via* APA [36]. In general, both AS and APA exhibit substantial tissue specificities. Therefore, in addition to transcription-determined gene expression, isoform variation serves as another layer of regulation, playing critical roles in cellular functions that shape phenotypic differences across tissues and organs.

4. Dysregulated RNA isoform variations in disease

As RNA isoform variation acts as a critical layer of gene regulation that is tightly controlled across different cell types and under different conditions, its dysregulation can disrupt gene functions and lead to diseases. In this section, we will mainly introduce isoform dysregulations in human genetic disorders and cancers. The aberrant splicing caused genetic disorders, can be classified into two classes, affecting cis-element responsible for appropriate splicing, and disrupting trans-factors regulating splicing such as components in spliceosome. The former includes mutations directly disrupting splice sites, accounting for an estimated 15% of human genetic disorders [37], as well as mutations that affect other splicing-related cis-elements. In total, it has been proposed that 50% or even 60% of human diseases are caused by these cis-element mutations [7]. For the mutations impairing trans-factors regulating splicing, an extensively studied example is spinal muscular atrophy (SMA). SMA is caused by mutations in the SMN1 gene, which affects around 1/4000 to 1/16,000 births worldwide [38]. SMN1 gene encodes SMN, a protein responsible for snRNP assembly, and thus its mutations should impair splicing globally. Compared to splicing, diseases caused by dysregulated polyadenylation are much less discovered. Still, studies reported several mutations disrupting PAS signal and causing hematological disorders [39].

Nevertheless, dysregulation for all three types of isoform variations has been observed in cancer. A study systematically quantifying promoter activities by analyzing 18,468 RNA-seq samples across 42 cancer types reveals widespread utilization of alternative promoters [8]. In line with the observation that active proliferated cells are preferentially expressing isoform with shortened 3′ UTR [36], 3′ UTR are globally shortened in cancer cells *via* APA compared to normal cells [40, 41]. Moreover, intronic polyadenylation (IPA), another type of APA that is located within the intron, is widespread in leukemia, which induces truncation of the encoded protein to inactivate tumor suppressor [42]. While the mechanism underlying widespread IPA is still under exploration, one of the main contributors of global 3′ UTR shortening in cancer cells is pointing to NUDT21 (CFIm25). To date, NUDT21 has been reported to regulate APA and contribute to cancer progression in glioblastoma [16], hepatocellular carcinoma [43], lung cancer [44], bladder cancer [45], and cervical cancer [46].

In addition to alternative TSS and APA, splicing has been much more extensively studied in cancer at both the DNA level and RNA level. Mutations disrupting canonical splice sites have been identified in various essential cancer-related genes, such as TP53 and BRCA1 [47], and this is a widespread mechanism for inactivating tumor suppressors [48]. Besides, recurrent somatic mutations in splicing factors have also been identified with representative studies showing frequent mutations in genes SF3B1, SRSF2, U2AF1, and ZRSR2 in hematopoietic malignancy, such as myelodysplastic syndromes (MDS) and leukemia [49–51]. A more recent study characterizing splicing factor mutations across 33 cancer types demonstrates that hotspot mutations of SF3B1 and U2AG1 are also frequent in multiple solid tumors as well [52]. Beyond mutations in splicing factors, MYC, a well-known proto-oncogene encoding a transcription factor, indirectly regulates splicing by promoting the expression of core spliceosome components as an essential step in lymphomagenesis [53]. These studies suggest potential high frequent splicing dysregulations in cancer. Indeed, comprehensive analysis of AS based on RNA-seq samples from 8705 cancer patients reveals more active AS in tumors compared to normal samples, as well as hundreds of aberrant splicing with novel exon-exon junctions that are not present in normal samples [54].

Taken together, these studies demonstrate the high frequency of dysregulated isoform variations in diseases, while aberrant splicing is the most evident. Many of these dysregulations disrupt gene functions by isoform switching and contribute significantly to pathogenesis. On the other hand, they may also serve as therapeutic targets for treatment. For instance, an antisense oligonucleotide drug modulating AS of gene SMN2 has been approved by the FDA for SMA treatment. Additionally, dysregulated isoform variations in cancer that induce novel ORFs such as splicing and IPA may serve as sources of neoantigens [55, 56], which are promising to be utilized for cancer vaccine development.

5. Technology advancement in quantifying and predicting isoform variations

The NGS is a technology that is capable of parallelly sequencing massive DNA fragments, up to hundreds of millions in one experiment. Applying NGS to complementary DNA (cDNA) libraries reverse transcribed from RNA, known as RNA-seq, has revolutionized gene expression profiling. In addition, RNA-seq is also efficient in detecting and quantifying alternative splicing events with reads (short fragment sequenced by the NGS) supporting splice junctions. An extensively used metric is the percentage of splicing in (PSI) that is calculated by reads supporting splicing in divided by the sum of reads supporting both splicing in and out, measuring the proportion of isoforms with splicing in. With this, global AS profiling has been performed across different tissues and species [57–59], as well as organs at different development stages [60].

As detecting and quantifying AS events from RNA-seq data are relatively straightforward, the computational methods for AS mainly focus on differential splicing analysis. rMATs and DEXSeq are two representative methods that have been widely utilized [61, 62]. However, accurate identification and quantification of alternative TSS and APA directly from RNA-seq data is more challenging compared to AS. To this end, various experimental methods have been developed based on TSS and PAS properties. We will briefly list these experimental methods together with the effects of computational approaches for accurate identification and quantification of TSS and PAS expression in Section 5.1. On the other hand, distinct cis-elements determine the definition and utilization of TSS, PAS, and splice site, endeavors have been conducted to predict them *in silico*, which involves both traditional machine learning technologies and more recent advancements in deep-learning-based artificial intelligence (AI), which will be highlighted in Section 5.2.

5.1 Identifying and quantifying alternative TSS and PAS from NGS data

There are two types of high-throughput experimental approaches for comprehensive TSS profiling. As mature transcripts transcribed by RNA polymerase II have a specific cap-like structure at the 5′ ends, cap analysis gene expression (CAGE) is a method capable of enriching 5′ ends of RNA. CAGE followed by massive parallel sequencing (CAGE-seq) is a high-throughput approach for transcriptome-wide TSS profiling [63]. Additionally, active promoter regions in chromatin are enriched with several specific histone modification markers, including tri-methylation on histone 3 lysine 4 (H3K4me3), acetylation on histone 3 lysine 9 (H3K9ac), and histone 3 lysine 27 (H3K27ac). The second type of method for inferring TSS utilization is based on chromatin immunoprecipitation (ChIP) assays with sequencing (ChIP-seq) for these three markers, even though with relatively lower resolution [64]. With CAGE-seq, the Functional ANnoTation of the Mammalian Genome (FANTOM) project identified 201,802 putative TSS across dozens of cell lines [65]. Among them, 70% (143,200) are from genic regions, while only 40% (56,793 out of 143,200) are associated with annotated transcripts based on GENCODE (**Figure 4A** and **B**), suggesting that the current transcript isoform annotation might be still not comprehensive. On the other hand, computational methods have also been developed to annotate and quantify TSS from RNA-seq data utilizing splice junctions across the first and second exons [8], or RNA-seq coverages together with sequence features [66].

For global PAS identification and APA quantification, dozens of experimental protocols have been developed. The majority of them are designed by enriching fragments of transcript 3′ end close to or comprising poly-A tail, such as 3P-seq, Aseq, PolyA-seq, and 3′ READS [67–70]. Accordingly, two widely used datasets have been constructed using data from these experimental 3′ end sequencing (3′ end-seq) approaches, including PolyASite and PolyA_DB [71, 72]. 53% of PolyASite (v2) PAS and 64% of PolyA_DB (v3) PAS are from genic region (**Figure 4C**). Even though the two databases are both obtained from 3′ end-seq data, the overlapped ones only account for 39% of the sites from PolyASite and 66% of the sites from PolyA_DB, suggesting the heterogenous of different 3′ end-seq protocols, for instance PolyA_DB uses the data from 3’ READS, while PolyASite uses the data from 3P-seq, Aseq, PolyA-seq et

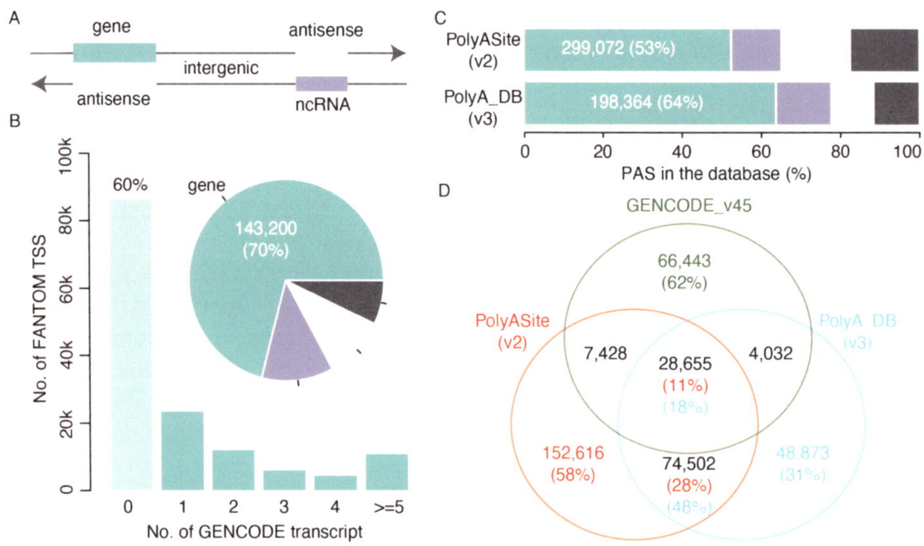

Figure 4.
Statistics of putative TSS and PAS identified by sequencing approaches from three databases. (A) The schematic shows the definition of four genomic regions based on the GENCODE annotation. (B) The pie chart shows the proportion of TSS across the four regions and the barplot illustrates the number of TSS associated with annotated transcript isoforms (distance <50 bp to the transcript start sites). (C) The proportion of PAS across the four regions. (D) Venn diagram showing the overlapped PAS across the two databases and GENCODE annotation. To be noted, the numbers in D and C are not consistent because multiple PASs might be merged together when calculating the overlap (distance <50 bp).

al. Moreover, 86% of PolyASite PAS and 79% of PolyA_DB PAS are not associated with any annotated transcript in GENCODE, again indicating the isoform annotation is far from complete (**Figure 3D**). In addition to experimental approaches, computational method for directly identifying PAS and quantifying APA from RNA-seq data are also feasible, while just the efficiency and accuracy are suboptionable. Almost all of them are designed by detecting drop points in RNA-seq coverages along the gene body, while many of them are only able to identify and quantify APA within 3′ UTR, such as TAPAS [73], QAPA [74], GETUTR [75], APAtrap [76], DaPars2 [77], and Aptardi [78]. Besides, IPAFinder is designed specifically for APA within intronic regions from RNA-seq data [61]. Nevertheless, we recently have developed APAIQ, an accurate method capable of transcriptome-wide APA identification and quantification from RNA-seq data, showing much higher precision and recall than previous methods [14].

5.2 Predicting isoform variations with DNA/RNA sequences

Owing to the heterogenous flexibilities of sequence features for TSS, PAS, and splice site, as well as their distinct pathogenic impacts, predicting the three types of isoform variations with DNA/RNA sequence are under different developmental stages and have different focuses. To date, there are many computational methods for predicting TSS but none of them is capable of predicting utilization of alternative TSS from the same gene. Hence, in this section, we will only focus on alternative polyadenylation and splicing. We will briefly introduce the historic computational methods and highlight the recent advancements utilizing artificial intelligence (AI) techniques in predicting these two kinds of variations.

5.2.1 Predicting PAS and APA

The early methods for PAS prediction mainly aim to discriminate true PAS from pseudo-ones that also comprises the PAS motif, *via* utilizing hand-crafted features from statistic frequency analysis [62, 79–81]. Thereafter, utilizing a set of latent sequence features extracted by Hidden Markov Models (HMM) trained with a benchmark dataset further significantly improves the accuracy [82]. These methods rely on a set of features based on prior knowledge or extracted by machine learning, which cannot capture the sequence information in full. With the advancement of deep neuron networks, sequences around PAS without further feature selection have been directly used as the input for deep learning models, which achieved good performance in binary classification of true/false PAS in multiple benchmark datasets [83, 84]. Still, they are not able to quantitatively predict the strength of each PAS, let alone the alternative usage across multiple PAS. To this end, we have developed DeeReCT-APA, a deep-learning architecture for predicting the usage of alternative PAS of a given gene [85]. However, DeeReCT-APA remains not feasible to evaluate strength of each PAS along the genome and predict mutation outcomes in APA. In 2023, using the large-scale PAS dataset from PolyA_DB, PolyAID achieved nucleotide resolution prediction of PAS along the genome. By optimizing the local gene structure of each PAS, PolyAID can predict its strength and usage. More importantly, applying PolyAID to scan the genome reveals thousands of genetic variants potentially impacting polyadenylation activity [86].

5.2.2 Predicting alternative splicing

Traditional computational methods for predicting splice events typically rely on motifs [87–89]. These methods assume the existence of characteristic sequences, or motifs, near splice acceptor and donor sites. Any mutations disrupting these motifs can consequently impact splicing events. While motif-based approaches offer intuitiveness and interpretability, they suffer from limitations in coverage and fail to fully capture the intricate regulatory mechanisms governing splicing. To overcome these limitations, some studies have integrated machine learning techniques, such as support vector machines and random forests, with splice event prediction [90–92]. While these traditional machine learning algorithms perform better than motif-based methods, they heavily rely on feature engineering, limiting their applicability and generalization.

SpliceAI pioneered the prediction of alternative splicing events through end-to-end deep learning models, utilizing gene sequences directly as inputs to estimate the probabilities of each position being an acceptor or donor site [93]. In comparison to predecessors such as MMSplice [94] and HAL [95], SpliceAI substantially extends the input sequence length to over 10,000 bases, facilitating the consideration of a broader range of information surrounding splice sites, especially regulatory elements around splice sites. To effectively process such extensive sequences, a residue-connected dilated convolutional neural network is employed. SpliceAI has exhibited remarkable performance in both splice site identification and the prediction of mutation impacts on alternative splicing events. However, SpliceAI lacks the capacity to differentiate between variations across different tissues and organisms, hindering its generalizability.

Several subsequent studies have endeavored to enhance performance based on SpliceAI, particularly in predicting the effects of mutations on alternative splicing. These efforts involve the integration of data from multiple species and multiple tissues [96], curated alternative splice sites [97], the scaling law [98, 99], and predictions from other tools [100]. Another approach to predicting splice events using deep learning models involves analogizing gene sequences to natural language text and training large language models on existing sequencing data to forecast splicing and mutation effects, as demonstrated by Enformer [101], DNABERT [102], and Hyenadna [103]. These methods rely on transformer-based architectures and large-scale sequencing data, which enable significant extension of the model's receptive field. For instance, Enformer achieves a receptive field of 100 kb and has demonstrated state-of-the-art performance on multiple gene expression prediction tasks. It is important to note that while these methods are designed for general gene sequence prediction tasks, they may not always perform optimally in predicting splice events.

Despite great progress in methods for identifying and quantifying alternative TSS, splicing, and polyadenylation from RNA-seq data, as well as deep-learning-based methods for predicting isoform variations with DNA/RNA sequence, they are all designed for detecting variations at the event level, rather than variations across different intact RNA isoforms. The TGS, from Pacific Bioscience (PacBio) and Oxford Nanopore Technology (ONT), which enable high-throughput sequencing of DNA or RNA with long read up to 25 kb and 300 kb, respectively, emerge as a powerful tool for full-length RNA isoform profiling. In 2022, a study implemented ONT to 88 samples from the genotype-tissue expression (GTEx) tissues and cell lines, revealing significant couplings between multiple alternative splicing events across isoforms and identified allelically specific utilization of isoforms [104]. This highlights the significance of utilizing full-length isoforms in assessing the outcome of genetic variants. Moreover, ~60% of TSSs captured by CAGE-seq and over 80% of PAS identified by 3′ end-seq data are not associated with any transcripts in GENCODE, suggesting the current isoform annotation is far from complete, raising the unmet needs for isoform identification with TGS data. With the accumulation of full-length isoform profiling data and the advancement of AI techniques, it is anticipated to see isoform centric deep-learning models that encompass all types of variation events and predict the outcome at the nature intact RNA molecular level.

DOI: http://dx.doi.org/10.5772/intechopen.1005044

Author details

Bin Zhang[1,2]* and Chencheng Xu[1,2]

1 Computational Bioscience Research Center, King Abdullah University of Science and Technology (KAUST), Thuwal, Saudi Arabia

2 Computer Science Program, Computer, Electrical and Mathematical Sciences and Engineering Division, King Abdullah University of Science and Technology (KAUST), Thuwal, Saudi Arabia

*Address all correspondence to: bin.zhang@kaust.edu.sa

References

[1] Olsen UD et al. Initial sequencing and analysis of the human genome. Nature. 2001;**409**(6822):860-921

[2] Venter JC et al. The sequence of the human genome. Science. 2001;**291**(5507):1304-1351

[3] Nurk S et al. The complete sequence of a human genome. Science. 2022;**376**(6588):44-53

[4] Harrow J et al. GENCODE: The reference human genome annotation for the ENCODE project. Genome Research. 2012;**22**(9):1760-1774

[5] Tilgner H et al. Deep sequencing of subcellular RNA fractions shows splicing to be predominantly co-transcriptional in the human genome but inefficient for lncRNAs. Genome Research. 2012;**22**(9):1616-1625

[6] Proudfoot NJ. Transcriptional termination in mammals: Stopping the RNA polymerase II juggernaut. Science. 2016;**352**(6291):aad9926

[7] Wang G-S, Cooper TA. Splicing in disease: Disruption of the splicing code and the decoding machinery. Nature Reviews Genetics. 2007;**8**(10):749-761

[8] Demircioğlu D et al. A pan-cancer transcriptome analysis reveals pervasive regulation through alternative promoters. Cell. 2019;**178**(6):1465-1477 e17

[9] Wang Z, Gerstein M, Snyder M. RNA-Seq: A revolutionary tool for transcriptomics. Nature Reviews Genetics. 2009;**10**(1):57-63

[10] Haberle V, Stark A. Eukaryotic core promoters and the functional basis of transcription initiation. Nature Reviews Molecular Cell Biology. 2018;**19**(10):621-637

[11] Lifton R et al. The organization of the histone genes in *Drosophila melanogaster*: Functional and evolutionary implications. In: Cold Spring Harbor symposia on Quantitative Biology. Cold Spring Harbor Laboratory Press; 1978. DOI: 10.1101/SQB.1978.042.01.105

[12] Cramer P. Organization and regulation of gene transcription. Nature. 2019;**573**(7772):45-54

[13] Proudfoot N, Brownlee G. 3′ non-coding region sequences in eukaryotic messenger RNA. Nature. 1976;**263**(5574):211-214

[14] Long Y et al. Accurate transcriptome-wide identification and quantification of alternative polyadenylation from RNA-seq data with APAIQ. Genome Research. 2023;**33**(4):644-657

[15] Xiao MS et al. Global analysis of regulatory divergence in the evolution of mouse alternative polyadenylation. Molecular Systems Biology. 2016;**12**(12):890

[16] Masamha CP et al. CFIm25 links alternative polyadenylation to glioblastoma tumour suppression. Nature. 2014;**510**(7505):412-416

[17] Matera AG, Wang Z. A day in the life of the spliceosome. Nature Reviews Molecular Cell Biology. 2014;**15**(2):108-121

[18] Turunen JJ et al. The significant other: Splicing by the minor spliceosome. Wiley Interdisciplinary Reviews: RNA. 2013;**4**(1):61-76

[19] Will CL, Lührmann R. Spliceosome structure and function. Cold Spring Harbor Perspectives in Biology. 2011;**3**(7):a003707

[20] Sheth N et al. Comprehensive splice-site analysis using comparative genomics. Nucleic Acids Research. 2006;**34**(14):3955-3967

[21] Yeo G, Burge CB. Maximum entropy modeling of short sequence motifs with applications to RNA splicing signals. RECOMB 03: Proceedings of the Seventh Annual International Conference on Research in Computational Molecular Biology. 2003. DOI: 10.1145/640075.640118

[22] Memczak S et al. Circular RNAs are a large class of animal RNAs with regulatory potency. Nature. 2013;**495**(7441):333-338

[23] Salzman J et al. Circular RNAs are the predominant transcript isoform from hundreds of human genes in diverse cell types. PLoS One. 2012;**7**(2):e30733

[24] Hansen TB et al. Natural RNA circles function as efficient microRNA sponges. Nature. 2013;**495**(7441):384-388

[25] Berg MG et al. U1 snRNP determines mRNA length and regulates isoform expression. Cell. 2012;**150**(1):53-64

[26] Almada AE et al. Promoter directionality is controlled by U1 snRNP and polyadenylation signals. Nature. 2013;**499**(7458):360-363

[27] Alfonso-Gonzalez C et al. Sites of transcription initiation drive mRNA isoform selection. Cell. 2023;**186**(11):2438-2455 e22

[28] Chan JJ et al. Pan-cancer pervasive upregulation of 3′ UTR splicing drives tumourigenesis. Nature Cell Biology. 2022;**24**(6):928-939

[29] Leppek K, Das R, Barna M. Functional 5′ UTR mRNA structures in eukaryotic translation regulation and how to find them. Nature Reviews Molecular Cell Biology. 2018;**19**(3):158-174

[30] Mayr C. What are 3′ UTRs doing? Cold Spring Harbor Perspectives in Biology. 2019;**11**(10):a034728

[31] Braunschweig U et al. Widespread intron retention in mammals functionally tunes transcriptomes. Genome Research. 2014;**24**(11):1774-1786

[32] Yan Q et al. Systematic discovery of regulated and conserved alternative exons in the mammalian brain reveals NMD modulating chromatin regulators. Proceedings of the National Academy of Sciences. 2015;**112**(11):3445-3450

[33] Gabut M et al. An alternative splicing switch regulates embryonic stem cell pluripotency and reprogramming. Cell. 2011;**147**(1):132-146

[34] Wong JJ-L et al. Orchestrated intron retention regulates normal granulocyte differentiation. Cell. 2013;**154**(3):583-595

[35] Brumbaugh J et al. Nudt21 controls cell fate by connecting alternative polyadenylation to chromatin signaling. Cell. 2018;**172**(1):106-120 e21

[36] Sandberg R et al. Proliferating cells express mRNAs with shortened 3 untranslated regions and fewer microRNA target sites. Science. 2008;**320**(5883):1643-1647

[37] Krawczak M, Reiss J, Cooper DN. The mutational spectrum of single base-pair substitutions in mRNA splice junctions of human genes: Causes

and consequences. Human Genetics. 1992;**90**:41-54

[38] Verhaart IE et al. A multi-source approach to determine SMA incidence and research ready population. Journal of Neurology. 2017;**264**:1465-1473

[39] Gruber AJ, Zavolan M. Alternative cleavage and polyadenylation in health and disease. Nature Reviews Genetics. 2019;**20**(10):599-614

[40] Xia Z et al. Dynamic analyses of alternative polyadenylation from RNA-seq reveal a 3′-UTR landscape across seven tumour types. Nature Communications. 2014;**5**(1):5274

[41] Mayr C, Bartel DP. Widespread shortening of 3′ UTRs by alternative cleavage and polyadenylation activates oncogenes in cancer cells. Cell. 2009;**138**(4):673-684

[42] Lee S-H et al. Widespread intronic polyadenylation inactivates tumour suppressor genes in leukaemia. Nature. 2018;**561**(7721):127-131

[43] Tan S et al. NUDT21 negatively regulates PSMB2 and CXXC5 by alternative polyadenylation and contributes to hepatocellular carcinoma suppression. Oncogene. 2018;**37**(35):4887-4900

[44] Huang J et al. Suppression of cleavage factor Im 25 promotes the proliferation of lung cancer cells through alternative polyadenylation. Biochemical and Biophysical Research Communications. 2018;**503**(2):856-862

[45] Xiong M et al. NUDT21 inhibits bladder cancer progression through ANXA2 and LIMK2 by alternative polyadenylation. Theranostics. 2019;**9**(24):7156

[46] Xing Y et al. Downregulation of NUDT21 contributes to cervical cancer progression through alternative polyadenylation. Oncogene. 2021;**40**(11):2051-2064

[47] Jayasinghe RG et al. Systematic analysis of splice-site-creating mutations in cancer. Cell Reports. 2018;**23**(1):270-281 e3

[48] Jung H et al. Intron retention is a widespread mechanism of tumor-suppressor inactivation. Nature Genetics. 2015;**47**(11):1242-1248

[49] Quesada V et al. Exome sequencing identifies recurrent mutations of the splicing factor SF3B1 gene in chronic lymphocytic leukemia. Nature Genetics. 2012;**44**(1):47-52

[50] Yoshida K et al. Frequent pathway mutations of splicing machinery in myelodysplasia. Nature. 2011;**478**(7367):64-69

[51] Graubert TA et al. Recurrent mutations in the U2AF1 splicing factor in myelodysplastic syndromes. Nature Genetics. 2012;**44**(1):53-57

[52] Seiler M et al. Somatic mutational landscape of splicing factor genes and their functional consequences across 33 cancer types. Cell Reports. 2018;**23**(1):282-296 e4

[53] Koh CM et al. MYC regulates the core pre-mRNA splicing machinery as an essential step in lymphomagenesis. Nature. 2015;**523**(7558):96-100

[54] Kahles A et al. Comprehensive analysis of alternative splicing across tumors from 8,705 patients. Cancer Cell. 2018;**34**(2):211-224 e6

[55] Ren X et al. Pervasive Intronic Polyadenylation Serves as a Potential

Source of Cancer Neoantigens. 2022. DOI: 10.21203/rs.3.rs-1537870/v1

[56] Li Z et al. An isoform-resolution transcriptomic atlas of colorectal cancer from long-read single-cell sequencing. bioRxiv. 2023 04.21.536771

[57] Wang ET et al. Alternative isoform regulation in human tissue transcriptomes. Nature. 2008;**456**(7221):470-476

[58] Merkin J et al. Evolutionary dynamics of gene and isoform regulation in mammalian tissues. Science. 2012;**338**(6114):1593-1599

[59] Barbosa-Morais NL et al. The evolutionary landscape of alternative splicing in vertebrate species. Science. 2012;**338**(6114):1587-1593

[60] Mazin PV et al. Alternative splicing during mammalian organ development. Nature Genetics. 2021;**53**(6):925-934

[61] Zhao Z et al. Cancer-associated dynamics and potential regulators of intronic polyadenylation revealed by IPAFinder using standard RNA-seq data. Genome Research. 2021;**31**(11):2095-2106

[62] Salamov AA, Solovyev VV. Recognition of 3′-processing sites of human mRNA precursors. Bioinformatics. 1997;**13**(1):23-28

[63] Shiraki T et al. Cap analysis gene expression for high-throughput analysis of transcriptional starting point and identification of promoter usage. Proceedings of the National Academy of Sciences. 2003;**100**(26):15776-15781

[64] Barth TK, Imhof A. Fast signals and slow marks: The dynamics of histone modifications. Trends in Biochemical Sciences. 2010;**35**(11):618-626

[65] The FANTOM Consortium and the RIKEN PMI and CLST (DGT). A promoter-level mammalian expression atlas. Nature. 2014;**507**(7493):462-470

[66] Zhou J et al. Annotating TSSs in multiple cell types based on DNA sequence and RNA-seq data via DeeReCT-TSS. Genomics, Proteomics & Bioinformatics. 2022;**20**(5):959-973

[67] Hoque M et al. Analysis of alternative cleavage and polyadenylation by 3′ region extraction and deep sequencing. Nature Methods. 2013;**10**(2):133-139

[68] Jan CH et al. Formation, regulation and evolution of Caenorhabditis elegans 3′ UTRs. Nature. 2011;**469**(7328):97-101

[69] Martin G et al. Genome-wide analysis of pre-mRNA 3′ end processing reveals a decisive role of human cleavage factor I in the regulation of 3′ UTR length. Cell Reports. 2012;**1**(6):753-763

[70] Derti A et al. A quantitative atlas of polyadenylation in five mammals. Genome Research. 2012;**22**(6):1173-1183

[71] Wang R et al. PolyA_DB 3 catalogs cleavage and polyadenylation sites identified by deep sequencing in multiple genomes. Nucleic Acids Research. 2018;**46**(D1):D315-D319

[72] Herrmann CJ et al. PolyASite 2.0: A consolidated atlas of polyadenylation sites from 3′ end sequencing. Nucleic Acids Research. 2020;**48**(D1):D174-D179

[73] Arefeen A et al. TAPAS: Tool for alternative polyadenylation site analysis. Bioinformatics. 2018;**34**(15):2521-2529

[74] Ha KC, Blencowe BJ, Morris Q. QAPA: A new method for the systematic analysis of alternative polyadenylation from RNA-seq data. Genome Biology. 2018;**19**:1-18

[75] Chang J-W et al. mRNA 3′-UTR shortening is a molecular signature of mTORC1 activation. Nature Communications. 2015;**6**(1):7218

[76] Ye C et al. APAtrap: Identification and quantification of alternative polyadenylation sites from RNA-seq data. Bioinformatics. 2018;**34**(11):1841-1849

[77] Li L et al. An atlas of alternative polyadenylation quantitative trait loci contributing to complex trait and disease heritability. Nature Genetics. 2021;**53**(7):994-1005

[78] Lusk R et al. Aptardi predicts polyadenylation sites in sample-specific transcriptomes using high-throughput RNA sequencing and DNA sequence. Nature Communications. 2021;**12**(1):1652

[79] Tabaska JE, Zhang MQ. Detection of polyadenylation signals in human DNA sequences. Gene. 1999;**231**(1-2):77-86

[80] Liu H et al. An in-silico method for prediction of polyadenylation signals in human sequences. Genome Informatics. 2003;**14**:84-93

[81] Cheng Y, Miura RM, Tian B. Prediction of mRNA polyadenylation sites by support vector machine. Bioinformatics. 2006;**22**(19):2320-2325

[82] Xie B et al. Poly (A) motif prediction using spectral latent features from human DNA sequences. Bioinformatics. 2013;**29**(13):i316-i325

[83] Xia Z et al. DeeReCT-PolyA: A robust and generic deep learning method for PAS identification. Bioinformatics. 2019;**35**(14):2371-2379

[84] Yu H, Dai Z. SANPolyA: A deep learning method for identifying Poly (A) signals. Bioinformatics. 2020;**36**(8):2393-2400

[85] Li Z et al. DeeReCT-APA: Prediction of alternative polyadenylation site usage through deep learning. Genomics, Proteomics & Bioinformatics. 2022;**20**(3):483-495

[86] Stroup EK, Ji Z. Deep learning of human polyadenylation sites at nucleotide resolution reveals molecular determinants of site usage and relevance in disease. Nature Communications. 2023;**14**(1):7378

[87] Desmet F-O et al. Human splicing finder: An online bioinformatics tool to predict splicing signals. Nucleic Acids Research. 2009;**37**(9):e67-e67

[88] Barash Y et al. Deciphering the splicing code. Nature. 2010;**465**(7294):53-59

[89] Cereda M et al. RNAmotifs: Prediction of multivalent RNA motifs that control alternative splicing. Genome Biology. 2014;**15**:1-12

[90] Dror G, Sorek R, Shamir R. Accurate identification of alternatively spliced exons using support vector machine. Bioinformatics. 2005;**21**(7):897-901

[91] Jian X, Boerwinkle E, Liu X. In silico prediction of splice-altering single nucleotide variants in the human genome. Nucleic Acids Research. 2014;**42**(22):13534-13544

[92] Mort M et al. MutPred splice: Machine learning-based prediction of exonic variants that disrupt splicing. Genome Biology. 2014;**15**:1-20

[93] Jaganathan K et al. Predicting splicing from primary sequence with deep learning. Cell. 2019;**176**(3):535-548 e24

[94] Cheng J et al. MMSplice: Modular modeling improves the predictions of genetic variant effects on splicing. Genome Biology. 2019;**20**:1-15

[95] Rosenberg AB et al. Learning the sequence determinants of alternative splicing from millions of random sequences. Cell. 2015;**163**(3):698-711

[96] Zeng T, Li YI. Predicting RNA splicing from DNA sequence using pangolin. Genome Biology. 2022;**23**(1):1-18

[97] Strauch Y et al. CI-SpliceAI—Improving machine learning predictions of disease causing splicing variants using curated alternative splice sites. PLoS One. 2022;**17**(6):e0269159

[98] Baeza-Centurion P et al. Combinatorial genetics reveals a scaling law for the effects of mutations on splicing. Cell. 2019;**176**(3):549-563 e23

[99] Wagner N et al. Aberrant splicing prediction across human tissues. Nature Genetics. 2023;**55**(5):861-870

[100] Rentzsch P et al. CADD-splice—Improving genome-wide variant effect prediction using deep learning-derived splice scores. Genome Medicine. 2021;**13**(1):1-12

[101] Avsec Ž et al. Effective gene expression prediction from sequence by integrating long-range interactions. Nature Methods. 2021;**18**(10):1196-1203

[102] Ji Y et al. DNABERT: Pre-trained bidirectional encoder representations from transformers model for DNA-language in genome. Bioinformatics. 2021;**37**(15):2112-2120

[103] Nguyen E et al. Hyenadna: Long-range genomic sequence modeling at single nucleotide resolution. Advances in Neural Information Processing Systems. 2024;**36**

[104] Glinos DA et al. Transcriptome variation in human tissues revealed by long-read sequencing. Nature. 2022;**608**(7922):353-359

Chapter 5

Perspective Chapter: Mastering RNA Interference (RNAi) Delivery – Strategies for Effective Targeting and Gene Silencing

Ahmed Kh. Abosalha, Stephanie Makhlouf, Paromita Islam, Shyam Mohapatra and Satya Prakash

Abstract

RNA interference (RNAi), a mechanism for post-transcriptional gene silencing using small interfering RNA (siRNA) or microRNA (miRNA), has emerged as a promising approach for managing numerous genetic disorders by selectively targeting and degrading the mRNA of implicated genes. However, the clinical application of these therapeutics is hindered by significant challenges that limit their delivery to target sites. RNAi therapeutics face multiple extracellular and intracellular barriers post-administration, including rapid glomerular excretion, recognition, and opsonization by the reticuloendothelial system (RES), and catalytic degradation by nucleases, leading to poor cellular and tissue penetration. To address these challenges, various delivery strategies have been explored to efficiently transport these RNAi therapeutics to their intended tissues. These strategies encompass chemical modification, bioconjugation with specific ligands, and carrier-mediated approaches. Nanotechnology-based delivery systems have demonstrated remarkable capabilities in encapsulating and delivering these molecules to their specific cells. Therefore, there is an urgent need to develop innovative delivery systems that can effectively encapsulate and target RNAi therapeutics. By targeting key genes, RNA interference holds the potential to address numerous genetic, viral, and cancer diseases at an early stage. This book chapter explores several studies detailing diverse design strategies aimed at overcoming the hurdles encountered in RNAi delivery.

Keywords: active drug-targeting, nanotechnology, RNA interference, gene silencing, liposomes

1. Introduction

Andrew Fire and Craig Mello received the Nobel Prize for their groundbreaking work on RNA interference (RNAi), a technique that holds immense promise for gene therapy in addressing various genetic disorders [1]. The identification of RNAi achieved a critical advancement in gene therapy, enabling scientists to elucidate the gene silencing mechanism and harness this new technology for gene function studies. Additionally, the progress in high-throughput screening and bioinformatics has enabled the targeting of several disease-causing genes, facilitating therapeutic applications and designing more effective personalized treatments. RNAi utilizes small siRNAs and miRNAs for post-transcriptional gene silencing by degrading the messenger RNA (mRNA) of targeted genes. Gene silencing through RNA interference (RNAi) takes place in the cytoplasm. Initially, a double-stranded RNA (dsRNA) is processed into smaller dsRNA fragments, called siRNAs and miRNAs by a Dicer enzyme. These RNAi molecules then bind to the Argonaute-2 (AGO2) protein, forming part of the RNA-Induced Silencing Complex (RISC). Within this complex, the RNAi duplex separates into two single strands: the guide and passenger strand. The passenger strand is degraded, leaving the guide strand to bind to complementary mRNA molecules. This binding leads to the destruction of the mRNA, preventing the translation of the target protein [2–4]. While siRNAs target specific mRNAs, miRNAs can affect multiple targets [5]. Few siRNA therapies have gained FDA approval for rare genetic disorders, such as hereditary variant transthyretin amyloidosis, acute hepatic porphyria, primary hyperoxaluria type 1, and hypercholesterolemia [6]. Despite RNAi's promising therapeutic efficacy, its clinical application faces hurdles, mainly due to challenges in delivering RNAi molecules to their intended sites. The delivery of siRNA therapies faces significant challenges due to barriers both inside and outside cells. These barriers include rapid clearance from circulation, susceptibility to degradation, limited cellular uptake, and rapid excretion through glomerular filtration. Researchers have explored various strategies to overcome these obstacles [3, 7, 8]. Chemical modifications enhance the stability and uptake of RNAi molecules, while bioconjugation with specific ligands enables targeted delivery to tissues of interest, reducing off-target effects. Nanotechnology offers promising solutions, with several proposed nanocarriers, facilitating the delivery of RNAi therapies to target cells, thereby improving their circulation time and reducing the need for frequent administration [4, 9]. These advancements aim to enhance the pharmacokinetics and efficacy of RNAi therapies. The current book chapter explores several RNAi delivery strategies aimed at improving the delivery of RNAi therapeutics for various gene-related disorders, demonstrating the potential of these approaches in advancing precision medicine.

2. Mechanism of action of RNAi therapeutics

Briefly, the process of gene silencing begins with the cleavage of long double-stranded RNA (dsRNA) by an endonuclease Dicer protein, resulting in the formation of small dsRNA fragments known as siRNAs or miRNAs. These small molecules then interact with the Argonaute-2 (AGO2) protein, a crucial component located at the center of a complex protein assembly called the RNA-induced silencing Complex (RISC). RISC identifies a group of diverse molecular complexes that can be directed to silence any gene. Typically, RISC activation occurs upon the detection of dsRNA within the cytoplasm of a eukaryotic cell [10]. This interaction leads to the separation of these duplexes into two strands: the passenger strand and the guiding strand. The complex formed by the guide strand and the RISC then recognizes and binds the complementary mRNA sequence of the target gene. This binding triggers the degradation of the targeted mRNA to small non-functional fragments, effectively silencing the translation process of the target protein as shown in **Figure 1**.

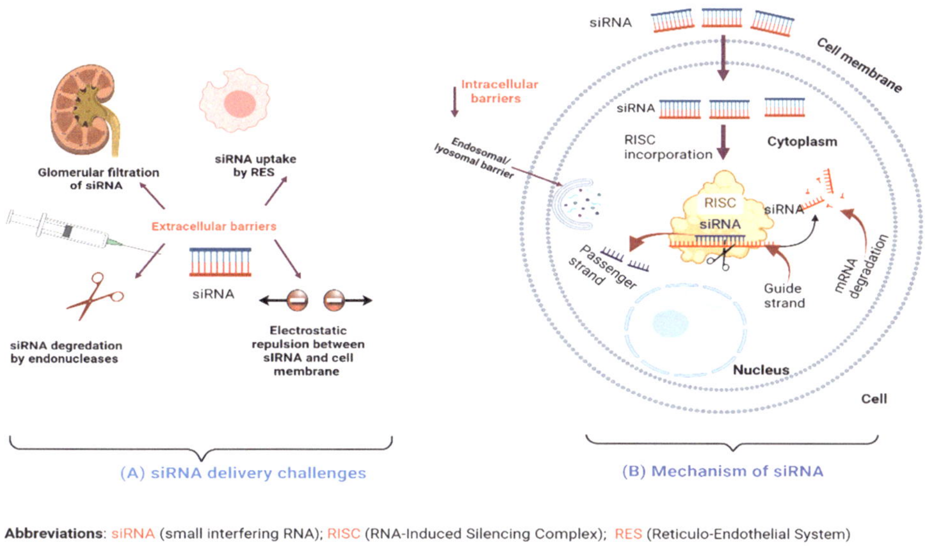

Figure 1.
Illustrative diagram showing the mechanism of action of RNAi therapies along with the challenges of their delivery to target sites. This figure was adapted from Abosalha et al. with permission [4].

3. Delivery barriers and limitations

RNAi is a regulatory mechanism found in most eukaryotic cells, serving as an efficient tool for post-transcriptional gene silencing. Their high specificity, selectivity, and potency give rise to promising targeted gene-specific inhibition. Its biochemical mechanism of action has rendered its clinical relevance across a wide spectrum of diseases such as infections, cancer, cardiovascular, and neurodegenerative disorders [11]. Yet, many intracellular and extracellular barriers disrupt the in vivo pharmacodynamics and pharmacokinetic profiles of naked unmodified RNAi molecules attributed to their poor absorption, unsatisfactory stability and distribution, rapid systemic clearance, and increased off-target effects [12]. Firstly, their anionic nature which is attributed to their phosphate backbone as well as their hydrophilic nature challenge their ability to be absorbed and to diffuse through the negative lipid bilayer membranes. Moreover, as soon as RNAi therapeutics are administered, they are susceptible to degradation by endonucleases, which cleave the phosphodiester bonds destabilizing these nucleic acids. Moreover, they can induce the secretion of inflammatory cytokines type I interferons (IFNs) since specific sequence motifs are recognized by pattern recognition receptors (PRRs) like toll-like receptors (TLRs) [7]. Interfering RNA are also subjected to phagocytosis through the reticuloendothelial system (RES) and to renal clearance due to their anionic surface charge and their small size and molecular weight. This poses an obstacle for this therapeutic RNAi to reach its target cells as its biodistribution and circulation time have been restricted. If not excreted by the kidneys or even the liver, the phagocyted RNAi up taken by non-targeted cells can lead to off-target effects and toxicity. Furthermore, following a successful uptake of RNAi into the targeted cell, it can also encounter intracellular challenges. While enclosed in endosomes, they face entrapment or experience a change of pH affecting the stability and half-life of these RNAi, reducing their effectiveness in gene silencing. Finally, among many intracellular components, RNAi must interact with the RNA-induced silencing complex (RISC) [13]. Some limitations may occur in this process depending on RNAi's delivery/loading pathway onto RISC, its structure's thermodynamic properties, and competition with endogenous RNA. These delivery barriers may interfere with the successful application of RNAi therapeutics and should be addressed efficiently to optimize the pharmacological efficiency of these therapies. For example, although 2'-OH modifications do not directly impact the RNAi machinery and potency, 2'-F modifications enhance the stability and half-life of siRNA. Chiu et al. demonstrated that the degradation of unmodified single-stranded antisense siRNAs is almost instantaneously, and the majority of these silencing RNA was undetectable within 30 mins. While duplex-siRNAs face a more sustained degradation, only 7% of siRNA remained after an hour. Conversely, 2'fluorinated double-stranded siRNA exhibited higher stability with around 68%–81% undegraded siRNA by the end of the experiment extending the persistence of RNA interference effects [14]. Another study showed that aptamer-conjugated siRNA enabled tumor-targeted siRNA delivery. STAT3 siRNA was specifically delivered to glioblastoma cells with the specific binding of the antagonist Gint4.T aptamer to the oncogenic receptor tyrosine kinase PDGFRβ. Enhanced specificity leads to increased cellular uptake of the bioconjugated siRNAs reaching 73% internalization in a glioblastoma cell line after an hour as reported by Esposito et al. [15]. Long et al. pursued another approach to combat breast cancer by loading siRNA-vascular endothelial growth factor (siVEGF) onto PAMPAM grafted halloysite nanotubes (PAMAM-g-HNTs). In vivo imaging showed the rapid excretion of freely intratumorally administered cys5-siVEGF by the mice. This obstacle was surmounted by the encapsulation of the cys5-siVEGF into the PAMAM-g-HNTs delivery system, where the majority of accumulation was seen in tumor sites. The observed enhanced permeability and retention (EPR) effect enables controlled gene release in the targeted tumor [16]. The above-mentioned examples highlight the integral role of the adopted strategies in effectively enhancing the biological activity of RNAi therapeutics. The reported delivery barriers are presented in **Figure 1**.

4. Strategies to overcome delivery barriers of RNAi therapies

The abovementioned barriers reveal that the design of a suitable delivery mechanism is essential for the effective clinical application of RNAi therapies. These delivery strategies should ensure the precise delivery of RNAi molecules to their intended target. Additionally, there is an essential demand for ongoing improvement of these strategies aimed at enhancing their targeting accuracy. Generally, three delivery strategies have been adopted to optimize the delivery of these therapeutics. The adopted techniques are chemical modification of naked RNAi molecules, bioconjugation with specific targeting ligands, and nanotechnology-based drug delivery systems (**Figure 2**).

4.1 Chemical modifications

The delivery of freely administered candidate RNAi is made feasible after undergoing chemical modifications. This strategy aims to mitigate the challenges arising from the original RNAi physicochemical properties. Mainly, the polyanionic phosphodiester skeleton of these molecules impinges the cell permeability and its cellular uptake as well as activates the RES leading to their opsonization followed by their rapid clearance [17]. Therefore, the masking of the negative charges along with the alterations of other characteristics such as hydrophilicity, its short structure, and sensitivity to ribonucleases

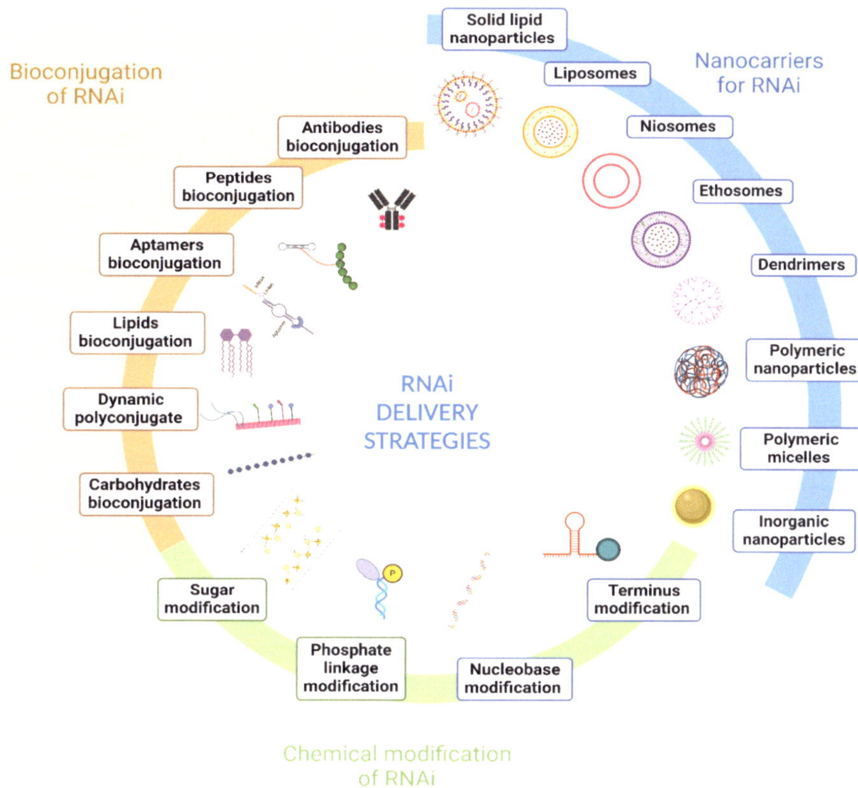

Figure 2.
Schematic diagram illustrating the adopted strategies to overcome the delivery barriers of RNAi therapeutics.

through chemical modifications may enable the oligonucleotide therapy to reach its target with an improved serum stability and biological half-life. Moreover, pattern recognition receptors (PRRs) recognize unmodified and unprotected RNAi molecules as foreign RNA, initiating the release of inflammatory cytokines and type I interferon (IFNs), which induces off-target interactions and toxicity [18]. Thus, for siRNA or miRNA to effectively exhibit their silencing effects, non-specific gene targeting must be reduced along with their immune-stimulatory activities, which are also further triggered by the RNAi nuclease-degradation byproducts. The main types of chemical modifications optimizing the chemical architecture of RNAi for clinical productivity are ribose modifications, phosphate modifications, and nucleobase modifications.

4.1.1 Ribose modification

A common and established approach of chemical modification is the addition of ribose moiety. Particularly, ribose modifications at the 2′ position have been widely explored as the 2’-OH group contributes, through hydrolysis, to the mechanism of endoribonucleases, hence RNAi cleavage [12]. Additionally, the 2’-OH group is not essential in RNAi silencing activity as it is not involved in the RISC, making this site a candidate target to be substituted with 2′-fluorine or 2′-o-methyl for enhancing properties of the oligonucleotide [11, 19]. Although 2’-OMe modification might decrease the activity of the sense strand by sterically blocking interactions, the conjugation of a fluorine group to the ribose moiety may compensate for this adverse effect by mimicking the 2'-OH group in size and charge [20, 21]. Overall, the alternating 2′F/2′OMe-RNA pattern offers increased thermodynamic stability, resembling that of a highly functional RNAi, as well as a higher binding affinity and half-life with a reduced immunogenicity [22, 23]. Alternatively, bicyclic and acyclic ribonucleoside substitutions may be used known as locked nucleic acids (LNA) and unlocked nucleic acids (UNA), respectively [12]. They introduce a chemical asymmetry into the RNAi duplex causing a conformation change promoting RISC loading of the guide strand, thus an increase of the RNAi activity and affinity [24].

4.1.2 Phosphate modification

Phosphate modifications are also used to enhance RNAi efficacy. Modifications with several phosphonate analogs at the 5′- end of the guide strand improve siRNA activity as it is essential for RISC recognition. Specifically, since following a 5′- ribose modification of the guide strand, mentioned above, the intracellular phosphorylation may be impacted, the chemical addition of a 5′-phosphate can rectify the activity of the RNA strand [25]. Furthermore, Lima et al. developed a phosphate analog more resistant de dephosphorylation in cells named 5′-(E)-vinylphosphonate (5′-E-VP), compelling for in vivo efficacy of RNAi on account of its suitable conformation and stereoelectronic properties [26]. Other phosphate modifications used in oligonucleotides include 5′-C-methyl analog, phosphorothioate (PS), and peptide nucleic acids (PNA) [23]. Particularly, phosphorothioate (PS) linkage primarily provides hydrophobicity reinforcing plasma protein binding tendencies, granting stability and an improved biodistribution, cellular uptake, and half-life circulation. However, it is important to note that high PS amounts may provoke chemical-related toxicities [12]. Hence, adequate numbers, positioning, and PS isomer, where the desired chirality for each strand ends is dictated by either the Sp or Rp configurations, are crucial for enhanced RNAi performance [27].

4.1.3 Base modification

Base modification has also been reported using nucleic acid analogs. While their use is limited, they contribute to a better understanding of gene silencing mechanism as well as prevent off-target effects [11, 23]. For example, according to Zhang et al. the activity of the passenger strand can be reduced with a 5′-nitroindole modification of the siRNA at position 15 of the passenger strand as a strategy to mitigate off-target effects without affecting the guide strand [28]. To enhance therapeutic effects, 5′-fluoro-2′-deoxyuridine substitution not only silences the targeted gene but also triggers cell death making it a candidate application for cancer therapy [29]. On the other hand, siRNA can be conjugated with fluorescent nucleobases such as 6′-phenylpyrrolocytosine to be used as in vivo monitors allowing for the visualization of siRNA internalization and other mechanisms [30].

4.2 Bioconjugation

The bioconjugation of RNAi therapies acts as an effective and promising approach for mitigating the shortcomings associated with delivering these molecules. Some of the commonly reported challenges such as vulnerability to endonucleases, limited cellular permeability, and inconsistent pharmacokinetic parameters may be addressed through their bioconjugation to specific ligands [31]. Literature reported a notable improvement in RNAi therapy's bioavailability, ability to target specific sites, stability in circulation, gene-silencing capability, and biological effectiveness because of their bioconjugation [3]. It is known that careful consideration of the conjugation site is crucial for determining the *in vivo* performance of the RNAi conjugates. Generally, the 5′ end of the guide strand, responsible for initiating RNA interference, and the 3′ end of the same strand are unsuitable for conjugation. Hence, the 3′ and 5′ ends of the passenger strand are preferred sites for bioconjugation. Moreover, bioconjugation to other sites like the 2'-OH group of ribose or nucleobases has also been explored [31, 32]. Several ligands have been investigated for their potential to overcome the delivery challenges of RNAi therapeutics as presented below:

4.2.1 Aptamers-RNAi bioconjugates

Artificial nucleic acid ligands, commonly referred to as aptamers, have risen as potent ligands for targeting numerous RNAi therapeutics. An aptamer stands as an artificially engineered, single-stranded RNA or DNA oligonucleotide, emerging as one of the most promising ligands for delivering RNAi therapeutics. These small three-dimensional oligonucleotide molecules exhibit remarkable specificity and high affinity toward a wide range of targets while remaining stable and adaptable to various chemical modifications. Aptamers pose additional advantages over other frequently used ligands for bioconjugation due to their low immunogenicity, high safety profile, cost-effectiveness, ease of synthesis, and extended shelf life. Based on these characteristics, aptamers serve as ideal delivery vehicles, imparting specificity, and selectivity to their conjugated molecules. Moreover, aptamers can efficiently enter cells via cell-mediated endocytosis, thereby overcoming poor cellular internalization of the delivered RNAi therapies and enhancing their cellular accumulation [33, 34].

4.2.2 Antibodies-RNAi bioconjugates

Generally, the antibody-drug conjugate approach holds considerable promise for targeted delivery of several drugs, peptides, nucleic acids, and genes. This technique of active drug targeting has got approval from regulatory authorities such as the FDA and EU for various cancer treatments [35, 36]. A variety of membrane receptors have emerged as crucial targets for therapeutic intervention in medical and pharmaceutical research. For example, antibodies designed to target overexpressed receptors on cancer cells, aim to disrupt the interaction between tumor and stromal cells, thereby impeding tumor progression and metastasis. Monoclonal antibodies targeting PD-1, PD-L1, and EGFR receptors have received approval for the treatment of various cancer types. Due to the high affinity and specificity of these ligands to their antigens, they are presently considered the conventional choice for bioconjugation for active targeting of RNAi therapies. Mostly, this conjugation method relies on the straightforward ionic attraction between positively charged antibodies and the anionic phosphate groups of RNAi molecules [3, 37].

4.2.3 Peptides-RNAi bioconjugates

Among various ligands of bioconjugation, cationic peptides have emerged as a promising strategy for the delivery of RNAi molecules owing to their facile synthesis, controllable dimensions, and adaptable structure for customizing physicochemical properties and specific targetability of conjugated therapeutics. Additionally, peptides can promote the cellular internalization of RNAi molecules due to shielding of their negative charge. Additionally, peptides can uphold a high degree of specificity and binding affinity to targeted receptors the same as antibodies. Moreover, their capacity to selectively bind specific proteins on cell surfaces, owing to their distinct tertiary structures, may be employed for the targeted delivery of siRNAs and miRNAs. The cyclic RGD (cRGD) peptide stands out as one of the most utilized peptides for this purpose [38, 39].

4.2.4 Lipids-RNAi bioconjugates

The incorporation of lipids into drug delivery systems has introduced significant advancements in delivery and targeting strategies. Unmodified RNAi molecules often face challenges due to their negative charge and hydrophilicity, hindering their optimal delivery to the desired tissue. Moreover, the hydrophilicity of RNAi therapeutics reduces their tendency to bind plasma proteins, making them suitable candidates for rapid glomerular excretion, resulting in a short half-life in circulation. Cationic lipids offer a potential solution by neutralizing the surface charge of these molecules, thereby enhancing their cellular permeability. The chemical composition of lipids significantly influences the effectiveness of RNAi delivery *in vivo*. For example, siRNAs conjugated with lipids such as cholesterol preferentially bind with LDL and predominantly accumulate in the liver. On the contrary, bioconjugation with lipids such as lithocholic acid exhibits a greater affinity for HDL and albumin, leading to deposition in various tissues including the liver, kidney, ovary, intestine, and others [40, 41].

4.2.5 Miscellaneous RNAi bioconjugates

Several studies reported the bioconjugation of siRNAs or miRNAs with other carbohydrate ligands such as glucose, galactose, lactose, and their derivatives. This bioconjugation showed an enhancement in the targeting, bioavailability, half-life, distribution, and pharmacological efficacy of encapsulated RNAi molecules [42, 43]. Additionally, small molecules can serve as highly specific and potent ligands for siRNA or miRNA delivery. The bioconjugation of RNAi to ligands such as folic acid and 2-[3-(1,3-dicarboxypropyl) ureido] pentanedioic acid (DUPA) could effectively target it to malignant cells overexpressing the respective folic acid receptor and Prostate-specific membrane antigen (PSMA) receptor, respectively. **Table 1** shows examples of RNAi therapies-bioconjugates for the management of different gene-related disorders.

4.3 Nanotechnologies

Nanocarrier systems have revolutionized drug delivery by offering innovative strategies aiming to harness the principles of nanotechnology to encapsulate RNAi. This allows these molecules to reach a wide range of applications with enhanced drug efficiency and minimal side effects. These nanoplatforms exhibit diverse characteristics based on their type, size, shape, and physical/chemical properties. Advanced nanocarriers like lipid nanoparticles and their derivatives including liposomes, lipid nanoemulsions, solid lipid nanoparticles, nanostructured lipid carriers, and lipid–polymer hybrid nanoparticles exhibit high biocompatibility when delivering encapsulated nucleic acids into the body. Other organic nanocarriers can be polymer-based such as PLGA and chitosan nanoparticles offering tunable sustained release of RNAi [53].

RNAi therapy	Conjugating ligand	Silenced gene	Targeted disease	Reference
3′-biotinyl-siRNA	The human insulin receptor-monoclonal antibody (HIR-MAb)	Luciferase	Neurological disorders	[44]
STAT3 siRNA	Humanized monoclonal antibody (Hu3S193)	Signal Transducer And Activator of Transcription 3 (STAT3)	Cancer therapy	[45]
siRNA	Anti-CD22 monoclonal antibody (Anti-CD22 Mab)	Glyceraldehyde-3-dehydrogenase (GAPD)	Lymphoma	[46]
Luc-siRNA	Cyclic- (arginine-glycine-aspartic) (cRGD)	luciferase gene	Melanoma	[47]
IRS1 siRNA	Insulin-like growth factor 1 (IGF1)	Insulin receptor substrate 1(IRS-1)	Breast cancer	[48]
IGF-1R siRNA	Mucin-1 (MUC1-apt)	Insulin-like growth factor receptor 1 (IGF-1R)	Metastatic breast cancer	[49]
Delta-5-desaturase siRNA	Epithelial cell adhesion molecule aptamer (EpCAM)	Delta-5-Desaturase (D5D)	Colon cancer	[50]
p-gp siRNA	Aptamer A6	P-glycoprotein transporter	Breast cancer	[51]
let-7 g miRNA	GL21.T Aptamer	let-7 g target genes	Lung cancer	[52]

Table 1.
Examples of RNAi therapies bioconjugation.

4.3.1 Solid lipid nanoparticles (SLNs)

Concurrent advancements in drug delivery involve lipid nanoparticles. They are the most commonly used carrier systems for RNAi encapsulation and delivery. SLNs are characterized by their amphiphilic properties encompassing hydrophilic head groups and hydrophobic tails [54]. These polar interactions enable the formation of a lipid monolayer or bilayer surrounding an aqueous core serving as a protecting environment for encapsulated payloads. Additionally, SLNs may be surface-modified with targeting ligands or PEGylation to enhance target-specific delivery and circulation time with the inhibition of RES uptake as well as inhibit SLNs aggregation [55]. Particularly, cationic SLNs, composed of ionizable cationic lipids or PEGylated lipids, are commonly used for nucleic acid delivery. 1,2-dioleoyl-3-trimethylammonium propane, also known as DOTAP, is one of the two most common cationic lipids [54]. When combined with DOPE in a 1:1 ratio, a reduction in toxicity is reported [56]. These nanoparticles are synthesized through high-frequency sonication between the lipid phase and the aqueous phase containing PEGylated surfactant [54]. The entrapment of the therapeutic RNAi is based on electrostatic interactions, which are also responsible for the controlled release kinetics of RNAi via endocytosis triggered by the contact of the positively charged cationic lipid and the negatively charged cell membrane [57]. Yang et al. have formulated a cationic lipid–polymer hybrid nanoparticle delivering siRNA toward breast tumor tissue for cancer therapy [58]. The cationic lipid monolayer, in which the siRNA was efficiently loaded via electrostatic forces, facilitated the carriage and escape of loaded siPlk1 into BT474 cells, inducing downregulation of the Plk1 oncogene and thereby cancer cell apoptosis. This hybrid nanoparticle shield with the cationic lipid is an attractive siRNA-delivering platform with significant potential in suppressing tumor growth and cancer therapies [58].

4.3.2 Liposomes

Liposomes are self-assembled amphiphilic lipid bilayers surrounding an aqueous core that may contain hydrophilic cargoes, including RNAi molecules. Its application range is further broadened with its ability to also encapsulate lipophilic and amphiphilic biologically active therapeutics. These lipid-based vesicles can be found as unilamellar, multilamellar, or multivesicular vesicles [59]. A common method of preparation involves oil-in-water emulsion where the lipids dissolved in organic solvent constitute the dispersion phase [59]. Their bilayer structure grants these carriers high biocompatibility and non-immunogenicity as well as stability and controlled release. Additionally, their ease of fabrication and customizable physicochemical properties promote cellular uptake and pharmacokinetics. Furthermore, optimized versions of traditional liposomes are being developed such as elastic liposomes (ELs) [60]. With the addition of surfactants, namely edge activators, ELs offer increased deformability and stress-dependent adaptability, enabling enhanced transdermal penetration for topical delivery targeting the efficient delivery of siRNA for the treatment of psoriasis and cervical carcinoma [61, 62].

4.3.3 Transferosomes

Transferosomes are a derivative of liposomes that are composed of edge activators. These vesicles are designed to particularly enhance the delivery of the payloads, including nucleic acid-based agents, across biological barriers such as skin or cell membranes [63]. These nanocarriers belong to the group of ultra-deformable hydrophilic vesicles characterized by their high malleability giving them the ability to deform and penetrate through narrow pores. In addition, the edge activators, which contain both lipophilic and hydrophilic moieties, enhance the diffusion of transferosomes through the skin via osmotic gradient activating via water evaporation [64]. Similar to liposomes, transferosomes are composed of lipid biomimetic bilayer, which supports their biocompatible and biodegradable properties. Moreover, anionic transferosomes could be employed as a strategy for mitigating foreign body reactions *in vivo* through the prevention of protein adsorption and immune system activation. Dorrani et al. reported that DOTAP/NaChol (6:1) transferosomes can penetrate the skin layer and effectively deposit BRAF-siRNA for the management of melanoma [65].

4.3.4 Ethosomes

Ethosomes are also ultra-deformable hydrophilic vesicles. They are composed of phospholipids, water, and a high content of ethanol ranging between 20 and 45%. Particularly, ethanol contributes to the formation of a highly elastic nanovesicle with improved deformability and fluidity enhancing skin absorption. Ethanol also increases the solubility of encapsulated drugs and imparts higher stability and smaller-sized non-aggregated vesicles attributed to the negative charge on the surface of ethosomes conferred by ethanol [66]. According to Chen et al. penetration enhancer such as SPACE-peptide can decorate the surface of cationic ethosomes optimizing the internalization of the DOTAP-SPACE-ethosomal system into epidermal keratinocytes [67]. The two conventional methods of preparation of ethosomes are the cold method and the hot method. The latter consists of heating the organic phase containing the phospholipids and the water phase to 40°C [66]. The final vesicles are obtained by either sonification or extrusion for both methods. Furthermore, additional alcohols such as propylene glycol (PG) and isopropyl alcohol can be included in ethanol-based vesicles forming binary ethosomes. These enhancers provide higher penetration and drug retention while penetrating the dermis layers. Also, as a humectant, PG aids with the hydration of the stratum corneum making it less susceptible to causing skin irritation or inflammatory [66].

4.3.5 Niosomes

Niosomes are non-ionic surfactant self-assembled vesicles. The amphiphilic surfactant consists of a polar and a non-polar group which allow for a specific orientation of the hydrophilic head toward the aqueous phase and hydrophobic tail shielded from water molecules. This configuration reduces the free energy at the interface, which effectively lowers the surface tension and facilitates the self-assembly of the niosomes [68]. Also, as an alternative to phospholipid-based carriers, niosomes present an enhanced *in vivo* stability against oxidation and degradation than phospholipids [69]. Additional advantages including high biocompatibility, permeability, encapsulation efficiency, and low production cost make niosomes potential candidates for commercialization [70]. The surface of these nanocarriers may also be decorated with hydrophilic polymer (e.g., PEG), cationic lipids (e.g., DOTAP), or conjugated with active targeting ligands/antibodies, among other modifications. For instance, Yang et al. developed a theranostic cationic niosome using a nonionic surfactant sorbitan monooleate (Span 80). This system efficiently mediated the intracellular delivery of siRNAs and miRNAs to human mesenchymal stem cells (hMSCs). A successful specific inhibition of miR-138 promoted osteogenic differentiation of hMSCs. In addition to RNAi delivery, this platform allows for cell labeling capabilities with the encapsulation of an amphiphilic dye, indocyanine green [68]. Alternatively, following the encapsulation of RNAi inside the hydrophilic core of niosomes, inorganic nanoparticles, such as superparamagnetic iron-oxide nanoparticles, can be entrapped within the niosomal barrier. Thereby, a targeted delivery via an external magnetic manipulation is achievable leading to an improved cellular uptake, as demonstrated by Maurer et al. on BT-474 cells for a breast cancer therapy [70].

4.3.6 Polymersomes

Polymerosomes are vesicular carriers formed by the self-assembly of amphiphilic copolymer blocks. The formed polymeric bilayer offers this nanoparticle distinctive properties for the delivery of encapsulated cargoes. The covalent crosslinking of the copolymer blocks leads to greater stability of the vesicle with the ability to modulate the membrane properties such as permeability, flexibility, and surface charge [71]. Also, the modification of the membrane surface is feasible for the conjugation of targeting ligands that present high binding affinity to proteins or receptors expressed on the surface of targeted cells. This active targeting enables selective drug delivery improving cellular uptake and minimizing off-target effects. Zheng et al. constructed a polymersome delivery system for the co-delivery of temozolomide (TMZ) and siRNA for the synergistic therapy of glioblastoma (GBM) [72]. The brain-targeted polymerosome is decorated with angiopep-2, a peptide that binds to the lipoprotein receptor-related protein-1 (LRP-1) receptor. As the latter is overexpressed on the surface of endothelial cells of blood-brain-barrier and GBM cells, this actively targeted nanocarrier showed an increased circulation time of siRNA/TMZ in the blood as well as an improved crossing of the blood-brain-barrier [72]. Alternatively, the polymersome membrane can be modified with stimuli-responsive moieties enabling the drug release rate to be programmable by external stimuli such as temperature, pH, and light [71].

4.3.7 Dendrimers

The term “dendrimer” originates from the Greek word “dendron,” signifying tree or branch. Dendrimers represent specially designed structured polymers characterized by their three-dimensional, extensively branched architecture, and uniformity in size and composition. Comprising a central core, branching arms, and functional groups at their terminals, dendrimers offer an ideal platform for drug delivery. Additionally, their internal structure provides a reservoir for drug encapsulation, while their surface can be decorated with diverse chemical groups, enhancing their targeting for specific clinical applications. Notably, dendrimers exhibit superior properties compared to conventional polymer-based delivery systems, including enhanced water solubility, excellent biocompatibility, and precise control over molecular weight. The utilization of dendrimers as a drug delivery system began to gain attraction in the late 1990s. They are typically synthesized via two methods: divergent and convergent synthesis. Divergent synthesis involves outward growth from the core, while convergent synthesis starts from the outer surface toward the core. Dendrimers offer advantages such as precise control over size and properties during synthesis, as well as the ability to attach various functional groups for specific targeting. They also exhibit prolonged circulation in the body, making them promising for delivering therapeutic molecules like RNAi therapeutics [73–75]. For instance, one study utilized a PAMAM dendrimer with a triethanolamine core to deliver Hsp27 siRNA to prostate cancer cells, demonstrating significant gene-silencing activity [76].

4.3.8 Polymeric nanoparticles

Polymeric nanoparticles have gained a special concern among all drug delivery techniques. These polymer-based nanocarriers showed interesting features as drug delivery vehicles. The ability to control the physicochemical characteristics of the formulated nanoparticles by controlling the selection and characteristics of utilized polymers has changed the landscape of drug delivery. Polymeric nanoparticles represent a class of polymer-based nanoscale structures that exhibit a uniform size distribution pattern. These nanoparticles show excellent biocompatibility and biodegradability, employing materials such as Poly-lactide co-glycolide (PLGA), Poly-lactic acid (PLA), Polycaprolactone (PCL), and chitosan. Their morphology, either nanocapsules or nanospheres exhibits heightened stability [77, 78]. Some of the commonly applied polymeric nanoparticles in drug delivery are discussed below.

4.3.8.1 PLGA nanoparticles

PLGA acts as a highly successful polymer in the encapsulation of several pharmacologically active molecules for medical applications. Its approval by the FDA for human administration underscores its exceptional biocompatibility and biodegradability. PLGA nanoparticles have gained significant interest in recent years owing to their versatility in transporting various types of drugs. Additionally, the capability to tailor their surface characteristics enhances their targeting and cellular internalization. PLGA nanoparticles were investigated across diverse therapeutic conditions, including vaccinations, chemotherapies, neurological disorders, inflammation, and other disorders. PLGA represents a meticulously studied biodegradable copolymer that undergoes degradation into non-toxic byproducts (H_2O and CO_2). PLGA nanoparticles degrade *in vivo* via hydrolysis of ester bonds to form monomeric anions (lactate and glycolate). PLGA is well-known for its ability to sustain the encapsulated drugs through a prolonged period. This sustained release profile extends the duration of action and decreases the frequency of administration of loaded drugs. Several methods were adopted to fabricate PLGA nanoparticles, including emulsion-solvent evaporation, double emulsion solvent evaporation, nanoprecipitation, salting-out, and supercritical fluid [79–81]. According to Cun et al. the encapsulation of small interfering RNA into PLGA nanoparticles, prepared by the double emulsion solvent evaporation method, may be optimized with the adjustment of the concentration of PLGA, the w/o phase ratio, the sonication time, quantity of loaded siRNA, and the acetylated bovine serum albumin (Ac-BSA) content in the inner water phase [82]. This strategy allows the obtention of high encapsulation efficiency of siRNA while preserving the negative particle zeta potential and small size. With a mean size of 220 nm and zeta potential of −7.3 mV, a hyaluronic acid-PLGA nanoparticle developed by Byeon et al. encapsulated paclitaxel (PTX) and focal adhesion kinase (FAK) siRNA with a 77–85% entrapment efficiency. The co-delivery of siRNAs permitted for the targeted delivery against chemoresistant ovarian cancer causing their apoptosis [83].

4.3.8.2 Glycogen nanoparticles

Glycogen is a natural hyperbranched polymer. It belongs to the polysaccharide class and is composed of glucose-repeating units connected by linear α-d -(1–4) glycosidic bonds and α-d -(1–6) branched chains [84, 85]. Glycogen-based nanoparticles are emerging as promising biocompatible and biodegradable delivery platforms. With a hydrodynamic diameter of 50 nm, these nanocarriers successfully accumulated in solid tumors via an enhanced permeability and retention (EPR) effect [85]. This cost-effective polymer is highly available since it is a renewable resource isolated from animals or plants. Similarly to other nanoparticles, glycogen's surface may be modified to confer anionic and hydrophobic properties using octenyl succinate (OS) groups for the delivery of antigens to dendritic cells [86]. Wojnilowicz et al. synthesized lactosylated glycogen-siRNA nanoparticles that demonstrated efficient targeting and penetration into 3D multicellular human prostate cancer spheroids which overexpress lectins [84]. A further optimization includes the engineering of the construct with pH-sensitive moieties using ethylenediamine (EDA). As the escape of RNAi from endosomes post-endocytosis is a limiting step in nucleic acid delivery, EDA enhances the proton sponge effect, promoting a more efficient endosomal escape of encapsulated RNAi and improving gene silencing effects [84].

4.3.8.3 Chitosan nanoparticles

Chitosan has gained attention as a promising natural biopolymer-based carrier in drug delivery owing to its biocompatibility, ability to adhere to biological surfaces, and capacity to enhance drug absorption. Nanoparticles formulated from chitosan and its derivatives typically exhibit a positively charged surface charge and possess mucoadhesive characteristics, enabling adhesion to mucous membranes and facilitating the sustained release of the encapsulated payload. Chitosan nanoparticles are characterized by their biodegradability, biocompatibility, low toxicity, and ease of preparation, introducing them as highly effective and promising in clinical applications. Moreover, chitosan nanoparticles can be readily functionalized to achieve targeted delivery and have received Generally Recognized as Safe (GRAS) status from the FDA. Unlike PLGA, The preparation of chitosan nanoparticles is conducted under mild conditions facilitated by chitosan's solubility in acidic aqueous solutions, eliminating the need for toxic organic solvents. These nanoparticles offer advantageous features in drug delivery for oral, ophthalmic, nasal, pulmonary, and transdermal delivery. Multiple methods are adopted

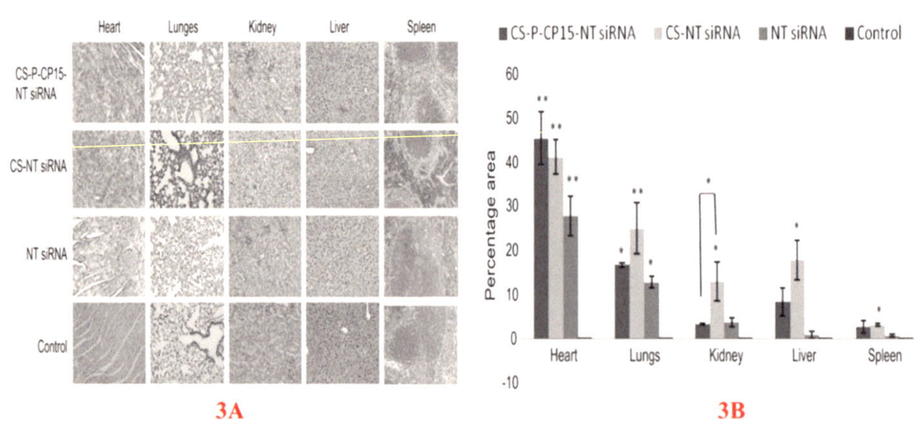

Figure 3.
The analysis of biodistribution of siRNA-loaded chitosan nanoparticles in various tissues 4 hrs after the administration of various formulations. ***Figure 3A*** *shows histopathological staining of the heart, lungs, kidney, liver, and spleen, administered at a dose of 0.5 mg/kg) CS-P-CP15-NT siRNA: chitosan-PEG-CP15, CS-NT siRNA: unmodified chitosan nanoparticles, NT-siRNA: non-targeting biotin-siRNA alone, and control as untreated.* ***Figure 3B*** *illustrates an image analysis of the mean percent area stained in the tumor tissues. This figure was adapted from Prakash et al. (US patent US 11,766,486 B2) with permission [90].*

for the fabrication of chitosan nanoparticles same as mentioned in PLGA nanoparticles preparation [87–89]. Prakash et al. prepared siRNA-loaded chitosan nanoparticles for the management of several types of cancer. The surface of the prepared nanoparticles was functionalized with TAT protein which enhances internalization and cellular uptake of the formulated siRNA nanoparticles. The results revealed the potential of the prepared siRNA-chitosan-TAT nanoparticles in targeting the encapsulated siRNA with a high concentration in different tissues [90] as shown in **Figure 3**.

5. Conclusion

The discovery of small interfering RNAi as therapeutic agents for gene silencing has generated considerable interest in the scientific community. RNAi shows significant promise for treating a wide range of diseases, including cancer, hepatic disorders, viral infections, and neurological conditions. Its efficacy in downregulating disease-associated genes and proteins has been demonstrated in various global health challenges. Few RNAi therapies have already been approved for clinical use, yielding remarkable outcomes. For instance, lumasiran has shown effectiveness in managing primary hyperoxaluria type 1 (PH1). However, delivering RNAi therapeutics to target tissues remains a significant challenge, limiting its effective application. Various strategies have been developed to address this issue, including chemical modifications to enhance RNAi molecules stability and biodistribution, bioconjugation with various ligands such as peptides and antibodies to improve cellular uptake and minimize adverse effects, and the use of nanotechnology-based carrier systems like liposomes, niosomes, dendrimers, solid lipid nanoparticles, and polymer-based nanoparticles to encapsulate RNAi and facilitate targeted delivery. The continuous optimization of appropriate strategies for RNAi therapeutics targeting is imperative to fully realize the therapeutic potential of this exciting therapeutic modality across various diseases.

6. Future of RNAi therapy

RNAi therapeutics may offer a novel approach to target numerous progressive genetic diseases by silencing their defective genes. They can also inhibit growth-promoting proteins in cancers, such as glioblastoma multiforme. Additionally, they may slow neurodegenerative diseases by targeting degenerative mediators, and treat viral infections by targeting virus mRNA. The COVID-19 pandemic has highlighted the potential of siRNA, particularly against the SARS-CoV-2 virus. Despite vaccine development, the emergence of viral variants always poses challenges. RNAi therapeutics can be potentially forwarded to silence viral gene expression and replication in various viral infections. Thus, advancing the delivery techniques of RNAi therapeutics is crucial for future therapeutic and vaccine development.

Acknowledgements

This work was supported by a grant from the Canadian Institute of Health Research (CIHR, grant 252743) to Satya Prakash. Ahmed Abosalha is fully funded by a scholarship from the Ministry of Higher Education of the Arab Republic of Egypt. The funders had no role in study design, data collection and analysis, decision to publish, or preparation of the manuscript. Paromita Islam is funded by the Islamic Development Bank Scholarship (2020-245622).

We thank the McGill University Imaging and Molecular Biology Platform (IMBP, Operetta High Content microscope) for equipment usage and services.

This research was funded by the US Department of Veterans Affairs Senior Research Career Scientist awards IK6BX1 and the NIH-RO1 -DK134000 provided to SSM. The views expressed in this article are those of the authors and do not necessarily reflect the position or policy of the Department of Veterans Affairs, or the United States government.

Conflict of interest

The authors declare no conflict of interest.

Author details

Ahmed Kh. Abosalha[1,2], Stephanie Makhlouf[1], Paromita Islam[1], Shyam Mohapatra[3] and Satya Prakash[1*]

1 Biomedical Technology and Cell Therapy Research Laboratory, Faculty of Medicine and Health Sciences, Department of Biomedical Engineering, McGill University, Montreal, Quebec, Canada

2 Faculty of Pharmacy, Pharmaceutical Technology Department, Tanta University, Tanta, Egypt

3 USF Center for Research and Education in Nano-Bioengineering, Department of Internal Medicine and James A Haley VA Hospital, Tampa, FL, USA

*Address all correspondence to: satya.prakash@mcgill.ca

References

[1] Watts G. Work on RNA Interference Brings Nobel Triumph. British Medical Journal Publishing Group; London; 2006

[2] Dana H et al. Molecular mechanisms and biological functions of siRNA. International Journal of Biomedical Science: IJBS. 2017;**13**(2):48

[3] Abosalha AK et al. A comprehensive update of siRNA delivery design strategies for targeted and effective gene silencing in gene therapy and other applications. Expert Opinion on Drug Discovery. 2023;**18**(2):149-161

[4] Abosalha AK et al. Clinical pharmacology of siRNA therapeutics: Current status and future prospects. Expert Review of Clinical Pharmacology. 2022;**15**(11):1327-1341

[5] Ahmadzada T, Reid G, McKenzie DR. Fundamentals of siRNA and miRNA therapeutics and a review of targeted nanoparticle delivery systems in breast cancer. Biophysical Reviews. 2018;**10**:69-86

[6] Zhang MM, Bahal R, Rasmussen TP, Manautou JE, Zhong X-B. The growth of siRNA-based therapeutics: Updated clinical studies. Biochemical Pharmacology. 2021;**189**:114432

[7] Wang J, Lu Z, Wientjes MG, Au JL-S. Delivery of siRNA therapeutics: Barriers and carriers. The AAPS Journal. 2010;**12**:492-503

[8] Whitehead KA, Langer R, Anderson DG. Knocking down barriers: Advances in siRNA delivery. Nature Reviews Drug Discovery. 2009;**8**(2):129-138

[9] Tatiparti K, Sau S, Kashaw SK, Iyer AK. siRNA delivery strategies: A comprehensive review of recent developments. Nanomaterials. 2017;**7**(4):77

[10] Pratt AJ, MacRae IJ. The RNA-induced silencing complex: A versatile gene-silencing machine. Journal of Biological Chemistry. 2009;**284**(27):17897-17901

[11] Alshaer W et al. siRNA: Mechanism of action, challenges, and therapeutic approaches. European Journal of Pharmacology. 2021;**905**:174178

[12] Hu B et al. Therapeutic siRNA: State of the art. Signal Transduction and Targeted Therapy. 2020;**5**(1):101

[13] Ly S, Echeverria D, Sousa J, Khvorova A. Single-stranded phosphorothioated regions enhance cellular uptake of cholesterol-conjugated siRNA but not silencing efficacy. Molecular Therapy-Nucleic Acids. 2020;**21**:991-1005

[14] Chiu Y-L, Rana TM. siRNA function in RNAi: A chemical modification analysis. RNA. 2003;**9**(9):1034-1048

[15] Esposito CL, Nuzzo S, Catuogno S, Romano S, de Nigris F, de Franciscis V. STAT3 gene silencing by aptamer-siRNA chimera as selective therapeutic for glioblastoma. Molecular Therapy-Nucleic Acids. 2018;**10**:398-411

[16] Long Z, Wu Y-P, Gao H-Y, Li Y-F, He R-R, Liu M. Functionalization of halloysite nanotubes via grafting of dendrimer for efficient intracellular delivery of siRNA. Bioconjugate Chemistry. 2018;**29**(8):2606-2618

[17] Juliano RL. The delivery of therapeutic oligonucleotides. Nucleic Acids Research. 2016;**44**(14):6518-6548

[18] Ali Zaidi SS, Fatima F, Ali Zaidi SA, Zhou D, Deng W, Liu S. Engineering siRNA therapeutics: Challenges and strategies. Journal of Nanobiotechnology. 2023;**21**(1):381

[19] Chernikov IV, Ponomareva UA, Chernolovskaya EL. Structural modifications of siRNA improve its performance in vivo. International Journal of Molecular Sciences. 2023;**24**(2):956

[20] Davis SM et al. 2′-O-methyl at 20-mer guide strand 3′ termini may negatively affect target silencing activity of fully chemically modified siRNA. Molecular Therapy-Nucleic Acids. 2020;**21**:266-277

[21] Manoharan M et al. Unique gene-silencing and structural properties of 2′-fluoro-modified siRNAs. Angewandte Chemie. 2011;**123**(10):2332-2336

[22] Khvorova A, Reynolds A, Jayasena SD. Functional siRNAs and miRNAs exhibit strand bias. Cell. 2003;**115**(2):209-216

[23] Dar SA, Thakur A, Qureshi A, Kumar M. siRNAmod: A database of experimentally validated chemically modified siRNAs. Scientific Reports. 2016;**6**(1):20031

[24] Doessing H, Vester B. Locked and unlocked nucleosides in functional nucleic acids. Molecules. 2011;**16**(6):4511-4526

[25] Khvorova A, Watts JK. The chemical evolution of oligonucleotide therapies of clinical utility. Nature Biotechnology. 2017;**35**(3):238-248

[26] Lima WF et al. Single-stranded siRNAs activate RNAi in animals. Cell. 2012;**150**(5):883-894

[27] Iwamoto N et al. Control of phosphorothioate stereochemistry substantially increases the efficacy of antisense oligonucleotides. Nature Biotechnology. 2017;**35**(9):845-851

[28] Zhang J, Zheng J, Lu C, Du Q, Liang Z, Xi Z. Modification of the siRNA passenger strand by 5-nitroindole dramatically reduces its off-target effects. Chembiochem. 2012;**13**(13):1940-1945

[29] Wu S-Y, Chen T-M, Gmeiner WH, Chu E, Schmitz JC. Development of modified siRNA molecules incorporating 5-fluoro-2′-deoxyuridine residues to enhance cytotoxicity. Nucleic Acids Research. 2013;**41**(8):4650-4659

[30] Wahba AS et al. Phenylpyrrolocytosine as an unobtrusive base modification for monitoring activity and cellular trafficking of siRNA. ACS Chemical Biology. 2011;**6**(9):912-919

[31] Tai W. Current aspects of siRNA bioconjugate for *in vitro* and *in vivo* delivery. Molecules. 2019;**24**(12):2211

[32] Schwarz DS, Hutvágner G, Du T, Xu Z, Aronin N, Zamore PD. Asymmetry in the assembly of the RNAi enzyme complex. Cell. 2003;**115**(2):199-208

[33] Kruspe S, Giangrande PH. Aptamer-siRNA chimeras: Discovery, progress, and future prospects. Biomedicine. 2017;**5**(3):45

[34] de Almeida CE, Alves LN, Rocha HF, Cabral-Neto JB, Missailidis S. Aptamer delivery of siRNA, radiopharmaceutics and chemotherapy agents in cancer. International Journal of Pharmaceutics. 2017;**525**(2):334-342

[35] Cortes JE et al. Prevention, recognition, and management of adverse events associated with gemtuzumab ozogamicin use in acute myeloid

leukemia. Journal of Hematology & Oncology. 2020;**13**:1-8

[36] Goldenson BH, Goodman AM, Ball ED. Gemtuzumab ozogamicin for the treatment of acute myeloid leukemia in adults. Expert Opinion on Biological Therapy. 2021;**21**(7):849-862

[37] Lee JW, Choi J, Kim EH, Choi J, Kim SH, Yang Y. Design of siRNA bioconjugates for efficient control of cancer-associated membrane receptors. ACS Omega. 2023;**8**(39):36435-36448

[38] Chernikov IV, Vlassov VV, Chernolovskaya EL. Current development of siRNA bioconjugates: From research to the clinic. Frontiers in Pharmacology. 2019;**10**:452642

[39] Shukla RS, Qin B, Cheng K. Peptides used in the delivery of small noncoding RNA. Molecular Pharmaceutics. 2014;**11**(10):3395-3408

[40] Wolfrum C et al. Mechanisms and optimization of *in vivo* delivery of lipophilic siRNAs. Nature Biotechnology. 2007;**25**(10):1149-1157

[41] Osborn MF et al. Hydrophobicity drives the systemic distribution of lipid-conjugated siRNAs via lipid transport pathways. Nucleic Acids Research. 2019;**47**(3):1070-1081

[42] Aviñó A et al. Synthesis and in vitro inhibition properties of siRNA conjugates carrying glucose and galactose with different presentations. Molecular Diversity. 2011;**15**:751-757

[43] Oishi M, Nagasaki Y, Itaka K, Nishiyama N, Kataoka K. Lactosylated poly (ethylene glycol)-siRNA conjugate through acid-labile β-thiopropionate linkage to construct pH-sensitive polyion complex micelles achieving enhanced gene silencing in hepatoma cells. Journal of the American Chemical Society. 2005;**127**(6):1624-1625

[44] Xia C-F, Boado RJ, Pardridge WM. Antibody-mediated targeting of siRNA via the human insulin receptor using avidin– biotin technology. Molecular Pharmaceutics. 2009;**6**(3):747-751

[45] Ma Y et al. Humanized Lewis-Y specific antibody based delivery of STAT3 siRNA. ACS Chemical Biology. 2011;**6**(9):962-970

[46] Palanca-Wessels MC et al. Anti-CD22 antibody targeting of pH-responsive micelles enhances small interfering RNA delivery and gene silencing in lymphoma cells. Molecular Therapy. 2011;**19**(8):1529-1537

[47] Alam MR et al. Multivalent cyclic RGD conjugates for targeted delivery of small interfering RNA. Bioconjugate Chemistry. 2011;**22**(8):1673-1681

[48] Cesarone G, Edupuganti OP, Chen C-P, Wickstrom E. Insulin receptor substrate 1 knockdown in human MCF7 ER+ breast cancer cells by nuclease-resistant IRS1 siRNA conjugated to a disulfide-bridged D-peptide analogue of insulin-like growth factor 1. Bioconjugate Chemistry. 2007;**18**(6):1831-1840

[49] Jafari R et al. Anti-mucin1 aptamer-conjugated chitosan nanoparticles for targeted co-delivery of docetaxel and IGF-1R siRNA to SKBR3 metastatic breast cancer cells. Iranian Biomedical Journal. 2019;**23**(1):21

[50] Xu Y et al. Specific delivery of delta-5-desaturase siRNA via RNA nanoparticles supplemented with dihomo-γ-linolenic acid for colon cancer suppression. Redox Biology. 2019;**21**:101085

[51] Powell D et al. Aptamer-functionalized hybrid nanoparticle

for the treatment of breast cancer. European Journal of Pharmaceutics and Biopharmaceutics. 2017;**114**:108-118

[52] Esposito CL et al. Multifunctional aptamer-miRNA conjugates for targeted cancer therapy. Molecular Therapy. 2014;**22**(6):1151-1163

[53] Zhang Y et al. Nanoparticle delivery platforms for RNAi therapeutics targeting COVID-19 disease in the respiratory tract. International Journal of Molecular Sciences. 2022;**23**(5):2408

[54] Dey AK et al. Tuning the immunostimulation properties of cationic lipid nanocarriers for nucleic acid delivery. Frontiers in Immunology. 2021;**12**:722411

[55] Zhu X et al. Surface De-PEGylation controls nanoparticle-mediated siRNA delivery *in vitro* and *in vivo*. Theranostics. 2017;**7**(7):1990

[56] Sun D, Lu Z-R. Structure and function of cationic and ionizable lipids for nucleic acid delivery. Pharmaceutical Research. 2023;**40**(1):27-46

[57] Mehta M, Bui TA, Yang X, Aksoy Y, Goldys EM, Deng W. Lipid-based nanoparticles for drug/gene delivery: An overview of the production techniques and difficulties encountered in their industrial development. ACS Materials Au. 2023;**3**(6):600-619

[58] Yang X-Z et al. Single-step assembly of cationic lipid–polymer hybrid nanoparticles for systemic delivery of siRNA. ACS Nano. 2012;**6**(6):4955-4965

[59] Šturm L, Poklar Ulrih N. Basic methods for preparation of liposomes and studying their interactions with different compounds, with the emphasis on polyphenols. International Journal of Molecular Sciences. 2021;**22**(12):6547

[60] Hussain A, Singh S, Sharma D, Webster TJ, Shafaat K, Faruk A. Elastic liposomes as novel carriers: Recent advances in drug delivery. International Journal of Nanomedicine. 2017;**12**:5087-5108

[61] Geusens B, Lambert J, De Smedt S, Buyens K, Sanders N, Van Gele M. Ultradeformable cationic liposomes for delivery of small interfering RNA (siRNA) into human primary melanocytes. Journal of Controlled Release. 2009;**133**(3):214-220

[62] Hattori Y, Date M, Arai S, Kawano K, Yonemochi E, Maitani Y. Transdermal delivery of small interfering RNA with elastic cationic liposomes in mice. Journal of Pharmaceutics. 2013;**2013**:149695

[63] Akram MW, Jamshaid H, Rehman FU, Zaeem M, Khan JZ, Zeb A. Transfersomes: A revolutionary nanosystem for efficient transdermal drug delivery. AAPS PharmSciTech. 2022;**23**:1-18

[64] Rajan R, Jose S, Mukund VB, Vasudevan DT. Transferosomes-a vesicular transdermal delivery system for enhanced drug permeation. Journal of Advanced Pharmaceutical Technology & Research. 2011;**2**(3):138-143

[65] Dorrani M, Garbuzenko OB, Minko T, Michniak-Kohn B. Development of edge-activated liposomes for siRNA delivery to human basal epidermis for melanoma therapy. Journal of Controlled Release. 2016;**228**:150-158

[66] Paiva-Santos AC et al. Ethosomes as nanocarriers for the development of skin delivery formulations. Pharmaceutical Research. 2021;**38**(6):947-970

[67] Chen M et al. Topical delivery of siRNA into skin using SPACE-peptide carriers. Journal of Controlled Release. 2014;**179**:33-41

[68] Lo CT, Jahn A, Locascio LE, Vreeland WN. Controlled self-assembly of monodisperse niosomes by microfluidic hydrodynamic focusing. Langmuir. 2010;**26**(11):8559-8566

[69] Paecharoenchai O, Teng L, Yung BC, Teng L, Opanasopit P, Lee RJ. Nonionic surfactant vesicles for delivery of RNAi therapeutics. Nanomedicine. 2013;**8**(11):1865-1873

[70] Maurer V et al. In-vitro application of magnetic hybrid niosomes: Targeted sirna-delivery for enhanced breast cancer therapy. Pharmaceutics. 2021;**13**(3):394

[71] Fonseca M, Jarak I, Victor F, Domingues C, Veiga F, Figueiras A. Polymersomes as the next attractive generation of drug delivery systems: Definition, synthesis and applications. Materials. 2024;**17**(2):319

[72] Zheng M et al. Brain-targeted polymersome codelivery of siRNA and temozolomide for effective glioblastoma chemo-RNAi synergistic therapy. ChemPhysMater. 2022;**1**(3):203-210

[73] An H, Deng X, Wang F, Xu P, Wang N. Dendrimers as nanocarriers for the delivery of drugs obtained from natural products. Polymers. 2023;**15**(10):2292

[74] Chauhan AS. Dendrimers for drug delivery. Molecules. 2018;**23**(4):938

[75] Wang J, Li B, Qiu L, Qiao X, Yang H. Dendrimer-based drug delivery systems: History, challenges, and latest developments. Journal of Biological Engineering. 2022;**16**(1):18

[76] Liu XX et al. PAMAM dendrimers mediate siRNA delivery to target Hsp27 and produce potent antiproliferative effects on prostate cancer cells. ChemMedChem. 2009;**4**(8):1302-1310

[77] Elmowafy M et al. Polymeric nanoparticles for delivery of natural bioactive agents: Recent advances and challenges. Polymers. 2023;**15**(5):1123

[78] Perumal S. Polymer Nanoparticles: Synthesis and Applications. Vol. 14. Wuhan, China: MDPI; 2022. p. 5449

[79] Rezvantalab S et al. PLGA-based nanoparticles in cancer treatment. Frontiers in Pharmacology. 2018;**9**:1260

[80] Loureiro JA, Pereira MC. PLGA Based Drug Carrier and Pharmaceutical Applications: The most Recent Advances. Vol. 12. Wuhan, China: MDPI; 2020. p. 903

[81] Alvi M, Yaqoob A, Rehman K, Shoaib SM, Akash MSH. PLGA-based nanoparticles for the treatment of cancer: Current strategies and perspectives. AAPS Open. 2022;**8**(1):12

[82] Cun D et al. High loading efficiency and sustained release of siRNA encapsulated in PLGA nanoparticles: Quality by design optimization and characterization. European Journal of Pharmaceutics and Biopharmaceutics. 2011;**77**(1):26-35

[83] Byeon Y et al. CD44-targeting PLGA nanoparticles incorporating paclitaxel and FAK siRNA overcome chemoresistance in epithelial ovarian cancer. Cancer Research. 2018;**78**(21):6247-6256

[84] Wojnilowicz M et al. Glycogen-nucleic acid constructs for gene silencing in multicellular tumor spheroids. Biomaterials. 2018;**176**:34-49

[85] Gálisová A et al. Glycogen as an advantageous polymer carrier in cancer theranostics: Straightforward in vivo evidence. Scientific Reports. 2020;**10**(1):10411

[86] Lu F, Mencia A, Bi L, Taylor A, Yao Y, HogenEsch H. Dendrimer-like alpha-d-glucan nanoparticles activate dendritic cells and are effective vaccine adjuvants. Journal of Controlled Release. 2015;**204**:51-59

[87] Jafernik K et al. Chitosan-based nanoparticles as effective drug delivery systems—A review. Molecules. 2023;**28**(4):1963

[88] Mohammed M, Syeda J, Wasan K, Wasan E. An overview of chitosan nanoparticles and its application in non-parenteral drug delivery. Pharmaceutics. 2017;**9**(4):53

[89] Garg U, Chauhan S, Nagaich U, Jain N. Current advances in chitosan nanoparticles based drug delivery and targeting. Advanced Pharmaceutical Bulletin. 2019;**9**(2):195

[90] Satya Prakash MM. Methods of Delivering Anionic Agents in Vivo Using Non-viral Nanoparticle-Based Delivery Systems, (in English). US Patent US 11,766,486 B2 Patent Appl. 17/069,701; USA; 2023

Chapter 6

The 2A Story: The End of the Beginning

Garry A. Luke and Martin D. Ryan

Abstract

Translational control of viral gene expression is a fundamental process essential for the vitality of all viruses. In special cases, signals encoded in the mRNA reprogram the ribosome to read the message in a different way, a process termed "translational recoding". The 2A region of the foot-and-mouth disease virus (FMDV) encodes a short sequence, only 18 amino acids, that mediates self-processing by a novel translational effect "ribosome skipping" rather than proteolysis. Briefly, 2A interacts with the ribosome exit tunnel to inhibit peptide bond formation at the C terminus of the 2A sequence. Translation terminates at this point, but then resumes elongation, creating a second independent protein product. Thus, discrete proteins can be produced from a single transcript. The 2A sequence is particularly useful in vector strategies (AAV and retroviral vectors) where the capacity to incorporate foreign DNA is limited. Use of 2A and "2A-like" peptides to link the sequences encoding several proteins in the same open reading frame has led to their increasing use as important tools in biotechnology and biomedicine. This technology has been crucial for the visual tracking of expressed proteins, human gene therapies targeting cancer, production of induced human pluripotent stem cells for regenerative medicine, creation of transgenic animals and plants and the improvement of CRISPR-Cas9 and TALEN genome editing methods.

Keywords: 2A peptide, mRNA translation, ribosome, ribosome skipping, recoding

1. Introduction

As obligate intracellular parasites with relatively limited coding capacity, viral strategies to sequester the host translation machinery target the initiation, elongation, and termination steps of protein synthesis. Although most translational control strategies operate at the rate-limiting initiation step, different regulatory mechanisms target elongation and termination. Commonly these involve translational control or "translational recoding" defined as instances in which "the rules for decoding are temporarily altered through the action of specific signals built into the mRNA sequences" [1, 2]. The two most common types of recoding elements program ribosomes to either shift the reading frame of an mRNA, typically by one base in either the 5′(−1) or the 3′(+1) direction (programmed ribosomal frameshifting) or reassign the "sense" of stop codons (UAA, UAG or UGA) leading to stop codon "Read-Through". Less common are recoding elements that cause ribosomes to bypass defined segments of mRNAs (ribosomal "hopping") or those that skip the synthesis of a specific peptide bond (ribosomal "skipping"). Ribosomal skipping, mediated by a "self-cleaving" 2A oligopeptide that manipulates the ribosome to "skip" the synthesis of the glycyl-prolyl peptide bond at its own carboxyl terminus leading to release of the nascent protein and translation of the downstream sequence. In this chapter we outline the development of this efficient methodology for the co-expression of multiple proteins from a single gene using a small 2A peptide originally identified in viruses.

2. Ribosome "skipping"

Among the five distinct types of picornavirus 2A proteins, a group of oligopeptide sequences collectively known as *Aphthovirus*-like 2A mediate a translational recoding event *in cis* known as "ribosome skipping", "StopGo" or "Stop Carry-on" translation [3–6]. Here a termination event occurs at a sense codon, followed by release of the nascent polypeptide and ribosomal translocation to the next in-frame codon. The function of the 2A sequence was first characterised from the positive-stranded RNA picornavirus Foot-and-Mouth Disease Virus (FMDV). The 2A oligopeptide is only 18 amino acids (aa) long (-LLNFDLLKLAGDVESNPG-), delineated by $3C^{pro}$ post-translational cleavage at its N-terminus and co-translational "cleavage" at its C-terminus [7–9]. The core sequence at the C-terminus of 2A is strongly conserved and contains the canonical motif D^{12}(V/I)E(S/T)NP$G_{2A}{}^{\downarrow}P^{19}{}_{2B}$ (where P^{19} refers to the completely conserved first residue of the downstream FMDV protein 2B). The less conserved part of the 2A sequence, located upstream of the motif, appears to be essential for 2A function [9, 10]. During this period the number of genome sequences was limited, but it was apparent that a similar motif was also present at the C-terminus of the longer cardiovirus 2A protein [11]. Analysis of recombinant FMDV polyproteins indicated FMDV 2A, together with the N-terminal proline of protein 2B, appeared sufficient for a co-translational "cleavage" between the upstream (capsid proteins) and downstream (RNA replication protein) domains of the polyprotein (-NPG$^{\downarrow}$P-) [7, 12]. Following cleavage, the 2A "tag" remains as a C-terminal extension of the upstream protein. The single proline at the N-terminus of the downstream protein confers a long half-life (>20 h) which should help increase protein stability [13]. Early studies showed the FMDV 2A region was not simply a substrate for a virus proteinase (L^{pro}, $3C^{pro}$), nor a substrate for a host-cell proteinase—"self-cleavage" was a novel translational effect [3, 7, 12]. Due to its mode of action within the ribosome the acronym CHYSEL (cis-acting hydrolase element) was proposed as an alternative name for 2A and 2A-like sequences to avoid confusion with protease mediated cleavage [14].

To monitor gene expression, artificial "self-processing" polyproteins were constructed with these 18 codons, plus the first aa (proline) of 2B (referred to as "2A"), separating green fluorescent protein (GFP—stop codon deleted) and β-glucuronidase (GUS) reporter-encoding sequences in a single open reading frame (ORF) encoding [GFP2AGUS] (**Figure 1**, pSTA1) [3, 15, 16]. In the absence of all other FMDV proteins, such artificial polyproteins comprised well-characterised, metabolically stable "reporter" proteins and used to program *in vitro* translation systems. These produced a simple translation profile that could be readily interpreted—and the accumulation of the processing products quantified. A control construct encoding [GFPGUS] produced only the fusion protein [GFPGUS], whereas

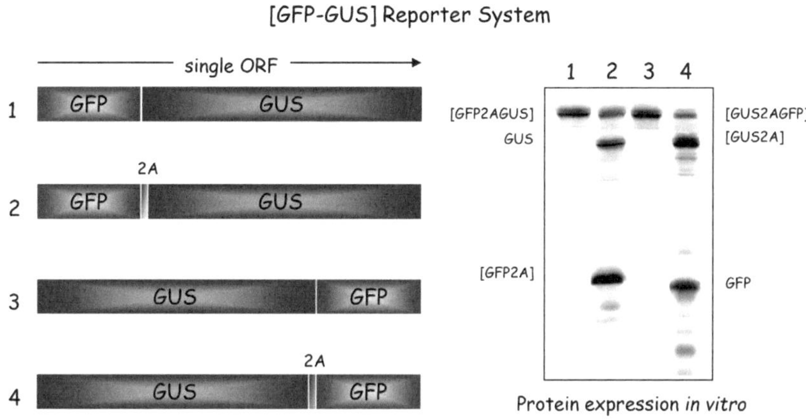

Figure 1.
Analysis of 2A-mediated "cleavage". *Artificial reporter polyproteins (boxed areas) used to programme in vitro translation systems are shown together with translation profiles obtained from rabbit reticulocyte lysates (right). The control pGFPGUS and pGUSGFP constructs produce only a single translation product—the [GFPGUS] and [GUSGFP] fusion proteins respectively. The translation profile from the pGFP2AGUS construct shows three major products: uncleaved [GFP2AGUS] and the cleavage products [GFP2A] and [GUS]. The profile from pGUS2AGFP also shows three major products: uncleaved [GUS2AGFP] and the cleavage products [GUS2A] and [GFP].*

the (GFP2AGUS) was shown to be highly active in mediating cleavage, producing the uncleaved polyprotein product (GFP2AGUS) (~5% of radiolabel incorporated) and the cleavage products (GFP2A) and [GUS], together accounting for ~95% incorporation of radiolabel. This approach gave the surprising result that the GFP reporter protein upstream of 2A accumulated to a higher level than that downstream of 2A (GUS) (**Figure 1**). Reversing the gene order (GUS2AGFP) produced the same type of imbalance. Having eliminated "trivial" causes for this imbalance (e.g. protein/RNA degradation, premature termination of transcription/translation) [3], these data were at variance with a proteolytic mechanism which predicts a unitary stoichiometry of the products. Inhibition of protein synthesis by the antibiotic puromycin produced a distinct product with a size corresponding to the upstream protein, indicating a pause on the mRNA at the site where the nascent chain is released [3]. The ribosome pause seen by ribosome toeprinting occurred at the end of the 2A coding sequence (-NPG↓P-), with glycine and proline in the P- and A- sites, respectively [17]. This imbalance was due to different levels of biosynthesis of each portion of the ORF and represents a novel type of recoding [5, 18].

3. Breaking the code

Owing to the degeneracy of the genetic code, a protein sequence can be encoded by many different synonymous mRNA coding sequences in protein biogenesis. Furthermore, many organisms, including viruses, tend to have biases towards certain synonymous codons (the "codon bias") in their genes. As described by Gao et al. [19] a marked codon bias within the FMDV genome is evident—the amino acids E, S, N, P, G, P tend to use GAG, TCC, AAC, CCT, GGG and CCC respectively. However, in the context of a synthetic reporter polyprotein, synonymous codon usage of this conserved motif does not affect apparent cleavage efficiencies whereas introducing non-synonymous changes impairs cleavage activity. Frameshifting the 2A oligopeptide with respect to the reporter proteins completely abolishes cleavage activity [3, 10, 15, 20]. Further, synonymous codon usage patterns for G_{2A} at the 2A/2B cleavage site (GGG, GGC, GGA, GGT) have no effect on the cleavage efficiency [19]. This supports the view that it is the amino acid residue rather than the nucleotide sequence which is critical for the activity of 2A. In contrast to these studies, Kjær and Belsham found that in FMDV genomes codon bias operates in encoding the NPGP motif, raising the possibility that the RNA sequence could also contribute to the recoding event [21]. It's noteworthy that conservative mutation of all potential nucleophilic amino acids within the highly conserved D^{12}(V/I)E(S/T)NP$G_{2A}{}^{\downarrow}P^{19}{}_{2B}$ motif are active—further proof that 2A-mediated cleavage is not a proteolytic mechanism [15]. The take home message from mutagenesis experiments is that 2A is largely intolerant to sequence alteration over most of its length—2A peptides are fine tuned to function as a whole [5, 9, 10, 15, 22]. Our own extensive mutagenesis indicates that several variations of the conserved motif still display some level of activity [10, 15]. However, certain 2A sequences have not evolved to produce a simple binary outcome. "Sub-optimal" 2A sequences usually result in either "standard" translation (generating a fusion protein), or, a molar excess of products upstream of 2A—due to dissociation of ribosomes after peptide release, rather than recommencing elongation. It is not difficult to imagine clear advantages associated with incomplete StopGo activity (e.g. dual protein targeting, described in Roulston et al. [23]), but also the possibility of "regulating" the ratio of up- to down-stream products (e.g. "sensor" of translational stress, described in [24]).

Various studies have demonstrated that synonymous codon usage bias plays an important role in the translation of certain mRNAs [25, 26]. While codon optimisation is routinely used to increase translational efficiency, with regard to 2A peptides, wild type sequences may be evolutionary optimised to enhance the StopGo mechanism. The length of the FMDV 2A used is also important for cleavage *in vitro*/*in vivo*—N-terminally truncated forms of 2A in our reporter system showed that the minimal length required for activity was 12aa (12 N-terminal and 1 C-terminal to the $G^{\downarrow}P$ site) [9, 15]. In the case of shorter 2As, cleavage efficiency has been improved by insertion of various spacer sequences immediately upstream of the 2A sequence such as a glycine-serine linker (e.g. -GSG- or -SGSG-, [27–29]; a 3XFLAG epitope tag -DYKDHDG-DYKDHDI-DYKDDDDK-, [30]; or a V5 epitope tag -GKPUPNPLLGLDST- [31]. These "flexible" linkers create a space between the N-terminal protein and the 2A peptide, favouring a conformation which facilitates efficient cleavage [32]. By contrast, an optimised Kozak sequence from the silkworm (*Bombyx mori*) placed immediately downstream of the 2A peptide, improved the expression of the sequence downstream of 2A [33]. Longer versions with extra sequences (>5aa) derived from the FMDV capsid protein ("1D") immediately upstream of 2A produce higher levels of cleavage [12, 15, 16]. After "tweaking" of the FMDV 2A sequence, 2A (+11aa 1D) proved to be the most favourable in terms of both length and cleavage efficiency [34, 35]. GSG linkers and longer versions of 2A sequences to improve "skipping" efficiencies are not fail-safe solutions and should be assessed empirically for every protein in context. Previously described position effects have also shown that expression of genes flanking 2A is highly dependent on their arrangement [33, 36–38]. For example, the yield of β-carotene by engineered yeasts could be altered by exchanging the order of codon-optimised carotenogenic genes *GGPPS*, *CARB* and *CARRP* [39].

4. A translational model of 2A

4.1 Reprogramming the ribosome

Based on dynamic molecular modelling and results from experiments with *in vitro* translation systems, the model of 2A-mediated translational recoding [3, 20, 40] proposes the nascent 2A peptide (~25aa) interacts with the exit tunnel of the ribosome such that the C-terminal portion is sterically constrained within a region of the peptidyl transferase centre (PTC) of the ribosome that cannot be accessed by prolyl-tRNA^{Pro}. The ribosomal PTC resides in the large ribosomal subunit and catalyses the two principle chemical reactions of protein synthesis: peptide bond formation and peptide release. It should be noted that the unique case of proline the nucleophile (nitrogen) is also sterically constrained since it is part of a ring structure. It has been shown that prolyl-tRNA^{Pro} is the poorest nucleophile among all aminoacyl tRNAs—polypeptide elongation is paused at this specific site. Our StopGo model predicts that (i) prolyl-tRNA^{Pro} dissociates from the A-site, (ii) the nascent polypeptide is released at this site by termination factors eRF1/3 and (iii) prolyl-tRNA^{Pro} (re) enters the ribosome a the A-site and must by translocated to the P-site to allow the next aminoacyl-tRNA to enter for resumption of translation and the synthesis of the downstream product (**Figure 2**) [17, 41]. Machida and colleagues showed however that processing of encephalomyocarditis virus proteins 2A and 2B in a reconstituted *in vitro* translation system requires neither eukaryotic initiation or termination (release) factors [42].

Our proposed model of this StopGo translational recoding event predicts that three alternative outcomes arise; having synthesised sequences upstream of 2A, ribosomes either (i) release the nascent peptide and then resume translation of the downstream sequences, (ii) release the nascent peptide and translation is terminated at that point, or, (iii) that no translational recoding occurs: the glycyl-prolyl peptide bond is formed and the protein is synthesised in the normal manner. The ratio of these translation products is dependent upon the specific 2A-like sequence in question—a view supported by the observations from many of the laboratories that have used StopGo protein co-expression applications. Initially studied in mammalian cell cultures (HeLa, [14]; HEK293, [43]; CHO, [11]) 2A-mediated ribosome skipping

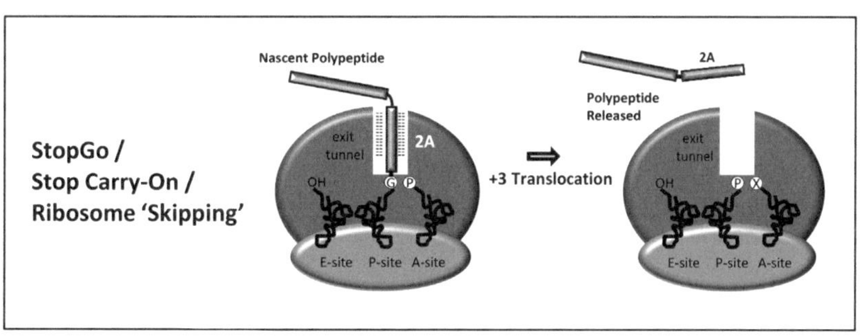

Figure 2.
Model of 2A translational "recoding" activity. *In ribosome "skipping", the 2A sequence is thought to interact with the ribosome exit such that the stereochemistry in the peptidyl transferase centre is altered: the peptide bond is not formed. The model proposes that prolyl-tRNA exits the A-site, eRF1/3 enters the A-site (at a sense codon) and terminates translation. After exit of eRF1, prolyl-tRNA then re-enters the A-site and is then (pseudo) translocated such that the A-site is now vacant and elongation can resume.*

functions in all eukaryotic expression systems tested to date: amoeba [45], fungi [38, 46–49], algae [50, 51], plants [52, 53] and animals [33, 54–56] but not prokaryotic systems: the structure of the ribosome and the exit tunnel is highly conserved among eukaryotes but differs between eu-and prokaryotes.

4.2 Targeted expression of recombinant proteins

Our model of the 2A mechanism predicted this "cleavage" would occur within the ribosome: that any protein downstream of 2A would emerge from the ribosome with a nascent N-terminus. Therefore, if one included a co-translational signal sequence immediately downstream of 2A, then this would be recognised by the signal recognition particle (SRP) as if it were generated during "normal" translation. In a proof-of-concept study this was the case: polyproteins were constructed comprising internal signal sequences and we were able to show that such proteins could be both co-expressed and independently targeted to sub-cellular sites (or secreted), greatly increasing the utility of the 2A co-expression system [57, 58]. To verify the applicability of this method to developmental studies, Trichas et al. designed a 2A bicistronic reporter that correctly processed a membrane-localised TdTomato gene (*Myr-TdTomato*) and nuclear-localised enhanced green fluorescent protein (EGFP) gene (*H2B-GFP*) in cell culture and transgenic mice [59]. Additionally, this approach produced functional expression of Myr-mCherry and H2B-GFP in the branchipod crustacean *Daphnia magna* [60]. Meanwhile, we demonstrated the (partially) active 2A-like sequences present at the N-terminus of a number of NOD-like receptor proteins (NLRs) within the purple sea urchin (*Strongylocentrotus purpuratus)* also play a dual role as exocytic pathway signal peptides. If 2A mediates translational recoding, the 2A signal sequence is synthesised as a discrete translation product separate from the downstream product which is localised to the cytoplasm. If 2A does not mediate translational recoding, the 2A signal sequence is fused to the downstream translation product, functions as a signal sequence and targets the fusion protein to the exocytic pathway—a novel form of dual protein targeting (**Figure 3**) [23].

4.3 The unwanted "tags"

The addition of partial 2A peptide sequences to the C-terminus of proteins may interfere with enzymatic activity [61]. For secreted proteins, inclusion of a furin recognition sequence (e.g. ↓-RRR-, ↓-RKRR-, ↓-RRKR-) between the first gene and 2A results in efficient removal of 2A residues—furin is a ubiquitous serine protease localised on the trans-Golgi networks of virtually all cell types [62]. Proteins expressed in plants/ fungi could have this tag removed by endogenous proteinases acting on similar hybrid linker peptides, LP4-2A in plants (SN↓AADEVAT) [63], TEV-2A in fungi (ENLYFQ↓S) [49]. Although not a full-proof solution, a GSG linker used in conjunction with a furin recognition site (e.g -furin-GSG-2A-, -GSG-furin-GSG-2A-) reportedly enhanced cleavage efficiency *via* increased exposure of the -RRKR- site [32, 44, 64]. The "unwanted" tag may remain—recognised by monoclonal antibodies, peptide epitopes can characterise, purify, and localise proteins of interest *in vitro* and *in vivo* [65, 66]. Commercial antibodies have been raised against the consensus 2A sequence, which thus serves as a useful target for identifying 2A-tagged proteins in biochemical assays—validated research applications include ICC, immunofluorescence, IP, and Western Blot [67, 68]. The presence of a proline amino acid residue (or often several additional amino acids, derived from restriction site sequences introduced during cloning) at the N-terminus

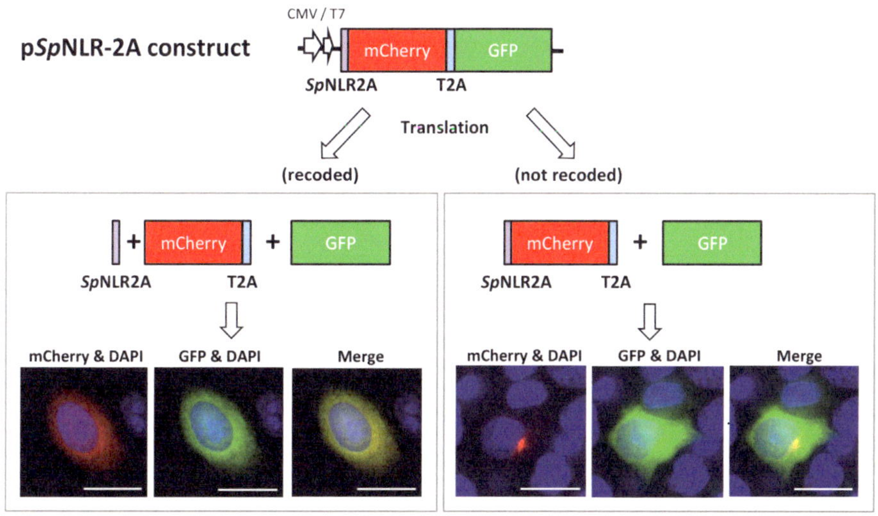

Figure 3.
Cleavage and signal sequence functions of 2A. *The wild-type and point mutant version was cloned upstream of sequences encoding cherry FP and GFP linked via Thosea asigna virus (TaV) 2A into a single ORF. Image analysis shows the wild-type 2A produces a high proportion of cherry localised in the cytoplasm (and diffuses into the nucleus). The mutant inactive 2A acts as a signal targeting cherry to the exocytic pathway (bars ~5µm. Nuclei stained with DAPI are shown in blue).*

of co-expressed proteins may affect protein stability within polycistronic constructs [69–71]. In this case, proteins that require authentic termini can be introduced at the first gene position.

5. 2A and 2A-like sequences

5.1 Viral and cellular 2As

The presence of 2A-like sequences has been reported in a number of viral genomes within different genera of the *Picornaviridae*, other positive strand viruses such as the *Dicistroviridae* and *Iflaviridae* [16, 72], double-strand RNA viruses belonging to the *Totiviridae*/*Reoviridae* families [73], and surprisingly in a tentatively assigned negative-sense single-stranded RNA virus of the *Bunyaviridae* family [72]. The positive-strand RNA viruses typically possess one 2A/2A-like sequence, but some viruses have two, three or more motifs—the picornavirus duck egg-reducing syndrome virus (DERSV) was shown to have a total of seven 2A proteins, the first six separated by the "DxExNPGP" sequence motif (**Table 1**) [74]. Translation *in vitro* with our pSTA1 dual reporter system [GFP-2A-GUS] shows some of these multiple $2A^{NPGP}$ sequences perform just as well as the commonly used FMDV 2A peptide: IMNV 2A1 and 2A2 [16]; Aalivirus A1/B1 2A1-2A4; Grusopivirus A1/C 2A1-2A3; Limnipivirus A1 2A1, B1 2A2, C1 2A1, D1 2A1-3; Mosavirus B1 2A1 and 2A2 (unpublished data). The advantage of releasing more than one protein from the same ORF suggests that host infection mechanisms in viruses with multiple 2A peptides in their genomes may be more complex [6]. Probing databases with this conserved motif revealed cellular 2A-like sequences within non-LTR retrotransposons (non-LTRs) of *Trypanosoma brucei*, *T. cruzi*, *T. vivax* and *T. congolense*, and, a range of simple aquatic species: *Xenopus tropicalis* (African

Genus	Species	$2A^{NPGP}$	Amino acid sequence	Accession no
Positive-stranded RNA viruses: *Picornaviridae*				
Aalivirus	AalV-A1	2A1	LLTSEGATNSSLLKLAGDVEENPGP	KJ000606
		2A2	FEMPYDDPEWDRLLQAGDIEQNPGP	
		2A3	PIPARPDPQWNNLQQAGDVEMNPGP	
		2A4	EHFNQTGGWVPDLTQCGDVESNPGP	
	AalV-B1	2A1	ATTLQVSEYLKDLTIDGDVESNPGP	MH453803
		2A2	LKVKKLEGDYVRDLTQEGVEPNPGP	
		2A3	SVRVTDAGWVRDLTVDGDVESNPGP	
		2A4	VFKCHDKCWVDDLTNCGDVESNPGP	
		2A5	IFKCHEGCWVEDLTVDGDVESNPGP	
	DERSV	2A1	TSTAQATSYVKDLTIDGDVESNPGP	UYL81882
		2A2	KTCREVEGSYVKDLTEEGIEPNPGP	
		2A3	LLKIGNAAWVRDLTEDGDVEENPGP	
		2A4	VYNCHESCWNRDLTIDGDVELNPGP	
		2A5	VFKCHEKCWQKDPTQDGDVEQNPGP	
		2A6	EFKCHEHCWVRDLTMDGDVEENPGP	
Avisivirus	AsV-A1	2A1	EVGAYDEVDHRDILMGGDIEENPGP	KC465954
		2A2	EMGVFDETDHRDILLGGDIEENPGP	
	AsV-B1	2A1	PQFEKERSAHEDVLLGGDVESNPGP	KF979333
		2A2	SESVQYLEPQIDICVCGDVERNPGP	
Grusopivirus	GrV-A1	2A1	FEKHVKPWRSQEDLSKEGIEPNPGP	KY312544
		2A2	ITDNRYKETDAKWLSRYGVEMNPGP	
		2A3	VTQDLYAATNQDQLSNQGIESNPGP	
	GrV-C	2A1	YFEERSPHPTQKELGQFGVETNPGP	MK443503
		2A2	ENNSNYDERDAKHLSRYGIEMNPGP	
		2A3	CVCTRWSPTMQSELGKYGIEKNPGP	
Kunsagivirus	KuV-C1	2A1	IAAASAQGWQRDLTQDGDVESNPGP	KY670597
		2A2	LGIVISDSVWQRDLPREGVEENPGP	
		2A3	SYDPLAPSQWCRDLTCEGIEPNPGP	
Limnipivirus	A1	2A1	CKEFVRESDNQELLKCGDVESNPGP	JX134222
		2A2	WDLSTGWFHFFRLLRSGDVEQNPGP	
	B1	2A1	MDVVDDYPFKRDLTRDGDVESNPGP	KF306267
		2A2	IDLVQAAYSRMRLLLSGDVEQNPGP	
	C1	2A1	KLLEQILAYKRDLTACGDVESNPGP	KF874490
		2A2	SRWIHARFARLRLLLSGDVEQNPGP	
	D1	2A1	EEEVDWGVGRMRLKMSGDVEENPGP	MG600094
		2A2	AVHLLVTWMRRRLTLSGDIESNPGP	
		2A3	DLRAVKSFIESQLMRAGDVERNPGP	
Mosavirus	B1	2A1	ESRGTGNCDATTISQCGDVETNPGP	KY855435

Genus	Species	$2A^{NPGP}$	Amino acid sequence	Accession no
		2A2	YVRRSANRTAADISQDGDVETNPGP	
Parechovirus	E	2A1	WFDARTGFKTPLMNPCGDVEENPGP	KY645497
		2A2	QIEKRYGYRFWLLMLCGDVELNPGP	
	RtPV	2A1	MLDRRMGYRSRILCQCGDVEENPGP	MF352429
		2A2	WFNKRSGYRSRLLSQCGDVEENPGP	
Potamipivirus	B1	2A1	LMEKTEEAGWLRDLTREGVEENPGP	MK189163
		2A2	FDDYHQEGGWIRDLTAEGVEPNPGP	
Unassigned	WCP	2A1	MKEDEAGGWKEDLTEDGDVESNPGP	MG00066
		2A2	EQAIPETTWRRDLTQSGDVESNPGP	
		2A3	PGAIPASVWVHDLTTDGDVESNPGP	
Unassigned	WP-LV 48	2A1	GPSCYDRNNHCNILLSGDIEENPGP	NC_032820
		2A2	VFNASYLDCFISLLSCGDIESNPGP	
		2A3	PIQGLTQRFESTLLLGGDIEENPGP	
Positive-stranded RNA viruses: *Iflaviridae*				
Iflavirus	EoPV	2A1	EQIVTAQGWAPDLTQDGDVESNPGP	NC_005092.1
		2A2	QRQNIIGGGQRDLTQDGDIESNPGP	
	PnPV	2A1	EQIVTAQGWVPDLTVDGDVESPNPG	NC_003113.1
		2A2	RRQNIIGGGQKDLTQDGDIESNPGP	
	DBMIV	2A1	EQIVTAQGWVADLTQDGDVESNPGP	NC_034384.1
		2A2	LRQNKILGGERDLTRDGDVESNPGP	
Non-segmented double-stranded RNA viruses: *Totiviridae*				
Unassigned	IMNV	2A1	IEISDCMLPPPDLTSCGDVESNPGP	
		2A2	IEKPFDKEEHTDILLSGDVESNPGP	

Table 1.
Multiple 2A/2A-like sequences in viruses.

claw-toed frog, vertebrate), *Branchiostoma floridae* (Amphioxus, Florida lancelet, cephalochordate), *Aplysia californica* (California sea slug, mollusc), *Crassostrea gigas* (Pacific oyster, mollusc), *Lottia gigantean* (Owl limpet, mollusc), *Nematostella vectensis* (sea anemone, cnidarian) and *S. purpuratus* (echinoderm) [75–77]. To allay public fears and bypass the use of animal-virus sequences, non-viral 2A variants (e.g. those found in the California sea slug and purple sea urchin) have been used just as effectively for coordinated multi-protein co-expression [78].

5.2 Comparison of active 2A sequences

Of the many 2A peptides identified to date, four viral 2As have been widely used in biotechnology and biomedicine: FMDV ("F2A"), equine rhinitis A virus (ERAV, "E2A"), porcine teschovirus-1 (PTV-1, "P2A"), and *Thosea asigna* virus (TaV, "T2A") (see **Table 2**) [27, 54, 59, 79]. Comparing the *in vitro* activity of different 2As inserted between GFP and GUS, $T2A_{20}$ has the highest cleavage efficiency followed by $E2A_{20}$, $P2A_{20}$ and $F2A_{20}$ [15]. In human cell lines, mice and zebrafish, cleavage and targeting

Virus	2A/2A-like sequence	Recoding activity	References
Picornaviridae			
FMDV ($F2A_{20}$)	-QLLNFDLLKLAG**DVESNPG**↓**P**-	***	[15, 34, 35]
FMDV ($F2A_{30}$)	-HKQKIVAPVKQLLNFDLLKLAG**DVESNPG**↓**P**-	****	[15, 34, 35]
ERAV (E2A)	-QCTNYALLKLAG**DVESNPG**↓**P**-	****	[27, 43, 45]
PTV-1 (P2A)	-ATNFSLLKQAG**DVEENPG**↓**P**-	****	[27, 43, 45, 64]
Tetraviridae			
TaV (T2A)	-EGRGSLLTCG**DVESNPG**↓**P**-	*****	[45, 65, 66]
The -DxExNPGP motif conserved among 2A/2A-like sequences is shown in red.			

Table 2.
2A/2A-like sequences most commonly used for protein co-expression.

of NLS-EGFP-2A-mCherry-CAAX was most efficient in $P2A_{19}$ linked constructs followed by $T2A_{18}$, $E2A_{20}$ and $F2A_{22}$ [43]. To test the performance of selected 2A peptides in insect cell cultures (*B.mori*) the cleavage efficiency of six types of 2A with a GSG linker were analysed: P2A, T2A, E2A, F2A, BmCPV2A and BmIFV2A. For the most used sequences $P2A_{22}$ exhibited the highest cleavage efficiency in all insect cell lines tested followed by $E2A_{23}$, $F2A_{25}$ and $T2A_{21}$ [32]. Interestingly, $P2A_{19}$ and $T2A_{18}$ functions in *Drosophila* are approximately equivalent both in cultured cells and *in vivo* [80]—given their poor efficiency at polypeptide separation, E2A and F2A may not be useful in *Drosophila* [80, 81]. A study to characterise the 2A system for metabolic engineering applications in *Saccharomyces cerevisiae* showed that the $F2A_{19}$, $T2A_{18}$, and $P2A_{19}$ sequences are functional in *S. cerevisiae* cells [82]—earlier analysis in *S. cerevisiae* indicated that ERBV-1 (Equine rhinitis B virus 1) 2A had the highest cleaving efficiency among 22 viral 2A sequences tested [48]. For potential upcoming amoeba-based bioprocesses codon optimised $P2A_{19}$, $T2A_{18}$, $E2A_{20}$ and $F2A_{22}$ were screened for activity in *Dictyostelium discoideum* [45]. In this work P2A and T2A performed the best with cleavage rates of 99.6% and 97.4% respectively, followed by E2A (95.5%), and F2A (66.9%). The availability of a range of 2A sequences can be useful—to minimise the risk of homologous recombination, it is wise to use different 2A peptide sequences if more than two genes are being linked.

6. IRES-dependent translation

Current strategies for multi-gene co-expression include: (i) pre-mRNA splicing; (ii) proteolytic cleavage sites; (iii) fusion proteins; (iv) IRESs (*i*nternal *r*ibosomal *e*ntry *s*ites); (v) self-cleaving 2A peptides and (vi) a new-kid-on-the-block termed HACKing (*H*ighly efficient and *A*ccessible system by *C*rac*King* genes into the genome) [83]. Among the six systems listed, the most popular strategies are 2A/2A-like sequences and viral IRES elements. Like the 2A peptide, the IRES was identified first among picornaviruses but in a different group, the *Enteroviruses*, typified by poliovirus (PV) [84]. Since then, IRES elements have been identified in other positive-sense RNA viruses such as encephalomyocarditis virus (EMCV) [85], DNA viruses [86, 87] and a growing number of cellular mRNAs involved in growth control, cell cycle progression and apoptosis [88]. In the majority of eukaryotic cells the mRNA 5′ 7meG "cap" is a signal for eukaryotic initiation factors (eIFs) to recruit ribosomes and initiate translation [89]. IRES elements allow the initiation of translation in a cap-independent manner, i.e., ribosomes bind internally without scanning the 5′ UTR of the transcript ensuring co-expression of genes before and after the IRES [90]. Most IRESs require IRES *trans*-acting factors (ITAFs) to function in addition to several canonical IFs [91]. These *cis*-acting RNA regulatory elements "hijack" ribosomes of the host cell, redirecting them towards the production of viral proteins [92, 93]. Viral IRESs have been classified into four different types based on their secondary structure and, in turn, their mechanism of initiation: *Type I* (enteroviruses/rhinoviruses), *Type II* (cardio-/aphthoviruses), *Type III* (flaviviruses e.g. HCV) and *Type IV* (dicistroviruses e.g. CrPV) [94, 95]. It has been shown that the efficiency of translation initiated from different IRES elements differs significantly [96–98].

Most IRES-based vectors developed up to now use picornavirus IRESs (e.g. EMCV and PV), based on the strong efficiency of such IRESs in transient transfection, compared to cellular IRESs [99, 100]. In mRNAs transcribed from bicistronic constructs, the first cistron is translated by a cap-dependent scanning mechanism while translation of the second cistron depends on the presence of IRES in the intercistronic space. The advantages of IRES-mediated systems include: complete separation of the coupled genes; lack of fusion proteins which may adversely affect the activity of the proteins; the relative expression of different genes can be "fine-tuned" by varying the strength of the IRES applied to each gene. IRES sequences, however, have limitations: (i) the large size (~500 bp) can reduce the packaging capacity in viral vectors [101], (ii) expression of the downstream gene can be as much as 10 fold lower than the upstream gene [102–104], (iii) recognition of different IRES elements varies with cell type, species, and even cell stress state [91, 97] and lastly (iv) the risk of homologous recombination and competition among different IRESs for translation factors [105].

Nevertheless, different IRES-based vectors including plasmids, adeno-associated virus (AAV)-derived and lentiviral vectors have been used successfully in pre-clinical as well as in clinical gene therapy protocols (reviewed in [106]). In plants, IRES-based constructs have been used to engineer pest resistance in tobacco [107], enhance salt and/or drought tolerance in potato [108] and produce carotenoids in rice endosperm [104]. However, compactness in length and their ability to allow the concatenated genes to be translated at equivalent levels both *in vivo* and *in vitro* has seen 2A peptides gain popularity over traditional IRES elements. Adenovirus [109], AAV [110], retrovirus [111], lentivirus [112] and plasmid [64] expression vectors incorporating 2A peptide sequences have been used in a variety of biotechnology and biomedical applications (reviewed in [113–115]).

7. Biotechnology/biomedical applications

7.1 Heterologous expression of multi-gene biosynthetic pathways in yeast

A particular advantage of using 2A co-expression technology is the ability to consistently express all the required genes in the same cell. For example, in biosynthetic pathways involving a number of separate enzymes it is critical they are all expressed in the same cell. If this is not the case, instead of progressing from reactants to products a breakdown in the pathway could lead to a build-up of volatile intermediates. Enzymatic systems requiring several cofactors have been reconstructed, by means of 2A peptides, both in *Pichia pastoris* and *S. cerevisiae* [48, 116, 117]. Significant advantages of the *P. pastoris* expression system include post-translational modifications such as glycosylation, proper protein folding and secretion (by Kex2 as signal peptidase) of recombinant proteins [118]. In the early days, environmental stress conditions imposed on the host presented a potential bottleneck in terms of recombinant protein production and secretion. Particular attention has been paid to the role of glycine betaine (GB) synthesis in abiotic stress resistance [119]. The GB pathway is a two-step oxidation from choline and betaine aldehyde, catalysed by choline monooxygenase (CMO) and betaine aldehyde dehydrogenase (BADH), respectively. The genes encoding the two enzymes of GB synthesis in the halophyte *Suaeda salsa* were cloned and fused with the F2A in a single ORF. The fused genes "*CMO-2A-BADH*" transformed in *P. pastoris* were expressed successfully and the polyprotein was cleaved to each functional protein [CMO-2A] and [BADH]. The recombinant yeasts were more tolerant to salt, methanol and high temperature stresses [120].

Biobased manufacturing for the production of fuels has become increasingly popular as the serious effects of global climate change become apparent. Using a viral 2A sequence, *P. pastoris* was engineered to produce the biofuels isobutanol and 3-methyl-1-butanol (3M1B, isoamyl alcohol). Upregulation of the endogenous L-valine biosynthetic pathway (*PpIlv5, PpIlv3, PpIlv6, PpIlv2*) and heterologous expression of the keto-acid degradation pathway (*LlkivD*, *ScADH7*) led to an engineered strain capable of producing isobutanol [121]. Specifically, the strain overexpressing all six genes produced a 100-fold improvement over the levels observed in the strains overexpressing only the two keto acid degradation pathway genes. In a follow on study, engineered strains overexpressing the keto-acid degradation pathway as well as the upper portion of the amino acid L-valine and L-leucine (*PpLeu1, PpLeu2, PpLeu6*) biosynthetic pathways were able to produce the platform chemical 3M1B [122]. Compared to the predominant biofuel ethanol, the advantages of 3M1B can be summarised as higher energy density, better miscibility with fossil fuels, lower water solubility, and greater applicability to conventional engines. The potential of this system is vividly demonstrated by the expression of nine genes from a single polycistronic transcript based on T2A peptides—presently, the construct with the highest number of genes expressed in a coordinated fashion. This expression strategy resulted in *P. pastoris* strains producing the target products of both the carotenoid (*CrtE, CrtB, CrtI,CrtY*) and violacein (*vioC, vioB, vioE, vioD, vioA)* biosynthesis pathways [47].

To date, a variety of studies have examined the use of multicomponent enzymatic systems based on the 2A approach in the baker's yeast *S. cerevisiae* [123–128]. The utility of 2A peptides has been demonstrated in several metabolic engineering applications, such as the production of C-glucosylflavones or β-carotene. Flavonoids are important phytochemical compounds with a range of medical benefits including powerful activities as antioxidants. In rice plants, two enzymes are responsible for the biosynthesis of flavone-C-glycosides, the cytochrome P450 flavanone 2-hydroxylase (F2H) and C-glucosyltransferase (CGT). While pathway engineering in tobacco resulted in minor C-glycoside formation, yeast transformed with the [F2H-F2A-CGT] polyprotein produced high concentrations of 2-hydroxynaringenin which could be converted chemically to the "nature-identical" plant product [129]. "Carotenoids" is a generic term used to designate a diverse group of pigments widely distributed in nature. Chemical synthesis of the flavour and fragrance (apo-) carotenoid β-ionone is economically impractical. For *de novo* production of apocarotenoids in yeast, three β-carotene biosynthesis genes from the carotenoid-producing ascomycete *Xanthophyllomyces dendrorhous* (*crtI*, *crtE* and *crtYB*) were co-expressed in *S. cerevisiae* from a single T2A polycistronic construct. To enable β-ionone production, a carotenoid-cleavage dioxygenase from raspberry (RiCCD1) was co-expressed in the β-carotene producing strain - a novel microbial production system for a fruit flavour compound [130].

7.2 Engineering carotenoid biosynthesis in plants

Conventional methods to "stack" transgenes in plants include sexual crossing, sequential re-transformation and single/multiple plasmid co-transformation [131]. These strategies, however suffer from the inherent weakness that co-expression of the heterologous proteins is unreliable. 2A/2A-like constructs have been successfully used to co-express β- and δ-zein proteins to improve the nutritional value of tobacco plants [132]; *mpi* (maize proteinase inhibitor) and *pci* (potato carboxypeptidase inhibitor) for insect and pathogen resistance in rice [133] and *Baccillus thuringiensis* (Bt) crystal proteins, Cry1Ab and Cry2Ab to delay insect resistance to Bt toxins in rice [134]. In a recent study, 11 genes were successfully introduced into transgenic maize to rebuild the anthocyanin biosynthesis pathway (*ZmBz1*, *ZmBz2*, *ZmC1* and *ZmR2*) by combining the advantages of a bidirectional promoter (BDP) and 2A linker peptides [135]. Carotenoids have attracted interest not only as a source of pigmentation but also for their beneficial effects on human health—since most animals are unable to synthesise carotenoids, they need to obtain them from food and dietary supplements. To alleviate vitamin A deficiency (VAD) through food intake, biofortified "Golden Rice" (*Oryza sativa*, GR) was engineered *via* two gene cassettes for the expression of the phytoene synthase (*Psy*) and carotene desaturase (*CrtI*) genes to produce β-carotene (provitamin A) (GR1 [136], GR2 [137]). Among GR varieties, "Korean Golden Rice" was developed using the recombinant *PAC* gene that linked the *Capsicum Psy* and *Pantoea CrtI* genes (PAC, *Psy-F2A-CrtI*) [104]. To increase the levels of carotenoids, the DNA sequences of these two carotenoid biosynthetic genes originating from heterologous sources, *Capsicum annum* for *Psy* and *Pantoea ananatis* for *CrtI*, were codon optimised for rice plants (*pstPAC*) [138]. In a separate study, Kim et al. genetically manipulated the carotenoid biosynthetic pathway in Korean soybean using an efficient *Agrobacterium*-mediated transformation method and the *PAC* recombinant gene to produce transformants whose β-carotene levels exceeded those reported in transgenic rice plants [139].

Zeaxanthin, capsanthin, canthaxanthin and astaxanthin are high-value carotenoids used industrially as colourants and feed supplements. Their antioxidant properties orchestrate important pathways in animals, including immuno/photo protection and oxidative stress modulation [140]. In both prokaryotes and eukaryotes, Astaxanthin is derived from β-carotene by hydroxylation and ketolation reactions catalysed by β-carotene hydroxylase (BCH) and β-carotene ketolase (BKT), respectively. In early studies of ketocarotenoid production, both genes from a marine bacterium (*Paracoccus* sp) were expressed simultaneously as a F2A polyprotein in both tobacco and tomato plants [141]. β-Carotene can typically be increased by the introduction of one or two transgenes, however producing diverse carotenoids beyond β-carotene (e.g. zeaxanthin and ketocarotenoids) typically requires the simultaneous engineering of a greater number of transgenes [142]. To produce downstream carotenoids, Ha and colleagues adopted three steps of the pathway to produce Zeaxanthin—a *BCH* expression cassette, under the control of the rice globulin promoter, combined with a *PAC* gene giving rise to a single T-DNA vector (pB-PAC; *Bch* and *Psy-2A-CrtI*). Astaxanthin was produced by the introduction of four steps (PSY, CRTI, BCH and BKT) using a single T-DNA vector (*pBAK-PAC*) with two cassettes for two bicistronic genes (BAK, *Bch-F2A-Bkt* and PAC, *Psy-F2A-CrtI*). The single T-DNA vectors resulted in the accumulation of zeaxanthin and astaxanthin in the endosperm of the transgenic rice seeds [143]. In a later study, bi-, tri and quadcistronic 2A systems for co-expression of these four genes were tested in transgenic rice seeds. To appease public concerns, three highly active 2A variants not found in mammalian viruses, $T2A_{20}$, $IMNV2A1_{30}$ and $IMNV2A2_{30}$ were used for the coordinated expression of multiple transgenes. This study demonstrated successful expression of two, three and four genes resulting in stepwise biosynthesis of β-carotene, zeaxanthin, adonixanthin and astaxanthin [144].

7.3 The broad utility of 2A and 2A-like sequences

Previous and more recent works employed the 2A approach to assemble biosynthetic pathways for heterologous expression in filamentous fungi. For bioproduct synthesis, the P2A peptide was employed to reconstitute synthesis of β-lactam antibiotics by moving the genes for the complete penicillin biosynthesis pathway from *Penicillium chrysogenum* (*pcbAB*, *pcbC*, and *penDE*) to the fungal host *Aspergillus nidulans* [145]. A similar approach was also used by Hoefgen and colleagues to produce the psychotropic mushroom alkaloid psilocybin by heterologous expression of the entire biosynthetic gene cluster (*psiH-psiD-psiK-psiM*) in *A. nidulans* [49]. A 2A peptide-based bicistronic protein expressing platform was used to monitor transgene expression (Cel7A, cellobiohydrolase) in the cellulase producing fungus *Trichoderma reesei* using eGFP as a marker (Cel7A-F2A-eGFP or eGFP-F2A-Cel7A) [38]. To date, 2A peptides have been used in various artificial reporter polyprotein systems comprising chloramphenicol acetyl-transferase (CAT), GUS and fluorescent proteins (FPs, e.g. GFP, RFP, YFP) in various cell types, as well as targeting to various subcellular localisations in plant [52, 146] and animal cells [56, 59]. Targeted endonucleases including zinc finger nucleases (ZFN), transcription activator-like effector nucleases (TALENs) and clustered regularly interspaced short palindromic repeats (CRISPRs) are increasingly being used for genome editing (GE) in numerous cell types and species. GE by using 2A peptide coupled co-expression of nuclease and fluorescent proteins combined with fluorescence-activated cell sorting (FACS) can aid selective enrichment of transfected cells. This approach to achieve higher genome editing efficiencies works well for these three major nucleases [147, 148]. To expand the experimental toolkit, antibiotic (hygromycin) and magnetic $H\text{-}2K^K$ cell selection methods have been developed to enrich transfected cells with ZFN/TALEN-induced mutations (2A-$Hygro^R$-eGFP and eGFP-2A-$H\text{-}2K^k$) [149]. In GE, the two colour "Traffic Light Reporter" (TLR; *eGFP-T2A-mCherry*) developed by Scharenberg and colleagues has proved invaluable for evaluating the two major DNA repair pathways, nonhomologous end-joining (NHEJ) and homologous recombination (HDR) [150]. Developing new methodologies governing CRISPR-Cas activity using 2A sequences include genetic switches [151], logic gates [152], and gene regulation circuits [153].

New types of cancer treatment *via* gene therapy promise to revolutionise management of the disease. Here, 2A is used to co-express the T-cell receptor TCRα and TCRβ chains (in transformed patient T-cells: *ex vivo* gene therapy) targeted against cancer antigens. Use of 2A sequences ensures both subunits of the receptor can be co-expressed at similar levels, minimising side effects. A second major impact in human health has been in the rapidly expanding field of regenerative medicine and transplantation. 2A has played a pivotal role in the co-expression of the multiple transcription factors required to produce induced pluripotent stem cells (iPSCs)—one can now make patient-specific stem cells relatively simply to avoid immune response problems and/or organ rejection (reviewed in [115]). Many other biotechnological applications that depend on the co-expression of genes use 2A/2A-like sequences e.g. the production of antibodies and antigens that can be used in vaccine production [64, 154, 155]. Bovine ephemeral fever virus (BEFV) is an economically important pathogen that causes an acute febrile illness of cattle and water buffalo in many parts of the world (Africa, the Middle East, Australia and Asia). Various studies have been conducted to develop an efficient vaccine for BEFV, including live attenuated, subunit and recombinant vaccines [156]. Although experimental and commercial BEFV vaccines have been developed, these suffer from either genetic instability, low efficacy, the need for multiple doses, or, are simply too expensive under field conditions. The 14.9 kb (−ve) ssRNA genome of BEFV contains 10 genes in the order 3′-N-P-M-G-G_{NS}-α1-α2-β-γ-L-5′ (**Figure 4**) [157]. G protein, as a class I transmembrane surface glycoprotein, is the target of neutralising antibodies and a prime candidate for subunit vaccine design [158]. In a recent study, we developed an antigen expression system to express recombinant G/G_{NS} glycoproteins with the transmembrane anchor domain deleted, enabling truncated proteins to be secreted into tissue culture media after mammalian cell transfection [65]. The V5 epitope tag was genetically fused to the C-termini of the proteins for protein detection and purification of expressed proteins from the cell media (**Figure 4**). Furthermore, a genetic fusion of each of the virus glycoproteins with GFP *via* T2A was used for live-cell fluorescence microscopy. In this "proof-of-principle" study, truncated G glycoprotein was detected throughout the exocytic pathway and secreted efficiently from BHK cells into the cell media. In a follow-on study we evaluated the immunogenicity of a secreted, C-terminally truncated form of bovine viral diarrhoea virus (BVDV) E2 glycoprotein in mice [66]. BVDV is the causative agent of one of the most widespread and economically important

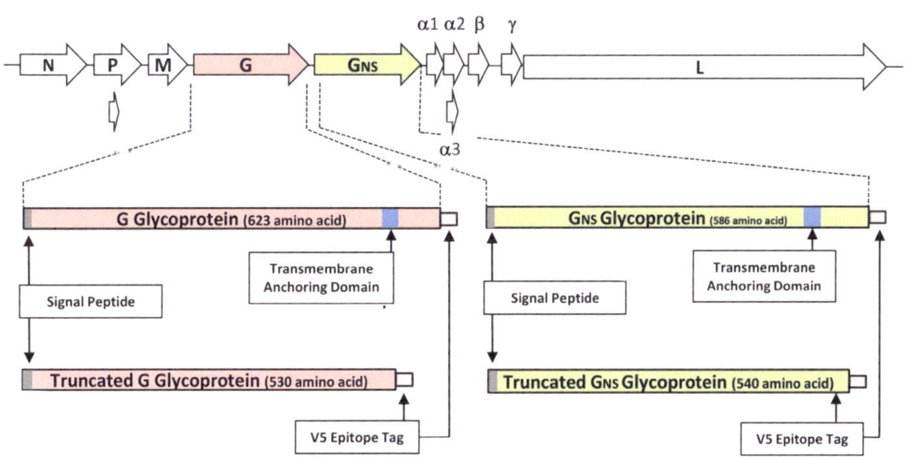

Figure 4.
Genome structure of BEFV and synthesis of the regions encoding the G and GNS glycoproteins. *Structural organisation of the BEFV genome shown as arranged in negative sense. The BEFV genome encodes five structural proteins including a nucleoprotein (N), a polymerase-associated protein (P), a matrix protein (M), a large RNA-dependent RNA polymerase (L) and a glycoprotein (G) spanning the viral envelope and a non-structural glycoprotein (G_{NS}) followed by a series of "accessory" proteins. Regions encoding the full-length G and G_{NS} proteins (boxed areas) are shown, together with the signal peptide (grey shaded areas) and the transmembrane anchoring domains (blue shaded areas). Regions encoding the C-terminally truncated (transmembrane anchoring domains deleted) forms of G and GNS proteins (boxed areas) are shown, together with the signal peptide (grey shaded areas) and the C-terminal V5 epitope tag (white boxes).*

virus infections in cattle [159]. Glycoprotein E2 plays a key role in host cell immune responses to viral infection [160]. Here, truncated E2 glycoprotein purified from cell media was found to induce both humoral and cellular immune responses in BALB/c mice. This antigen expression system provides both a simple purification protocol along with a feasible strategy for further, large-scale, production of vaccines.

A particularly useful aspect of the ribosome skipping mechanism is the possibility of differentially targeting the proteins produced from a single gene. For example, Park and colleagues used three 2A peptides (F2A, T2A and E2A) to simultaneously express four distinct fluorescent protein variants targeted to subcellular compartments such as mitochondria, nuclei, endosomes, and membranes for real-time monitoring of cellular dynamics in HeLa cells [161]. To facilitate studies of subcellular Ca^{2+} signalling in insulin-secreting pancreatic beta cells, particularly, signalling between the ER and mitochondria, Jeyarajan et al. [162] designed a plasmid that contained the sequences of two different Ca^{2+} reporter molecules, G-CEPIA-er and R-CEPIA3-mt, separated by T2A. Successful segregation of the two probes to their respective organelles allowed simultaneous measurement of changes in free Ca^{2+} to be made using live cell imaging in real time. 2A peptides were also used for the co-expression and differential subcellular targeting of two fluorescent marker proteins in insect cell culture systems (*Drosophila melanogaster* S2 cells) and *Drosophila suzukii* cell lines [163]. All four 2A peptides tested ($F2A_{31}$, $F2A_{32}$, T2A, DCV2A) showed comparable activity in cell lines, leading to the production of independent upstream and downstream proteins that were directed to the nucleus or membrane by a C-terminal nuclear localisation signal (NLS) on the upstream protein and a poly-lysine/CAAX membrane anchor on the downstream protein.

8. Conclusions

In prokaryotes proteins with linked functions (e.g. the formation of macromolecular structures, biochemical pathways) can be expressed in a co-ordinated manner by encoding multiple proteins as polycistronic mRNAs: a single RNA is transcribed from different genes organised—concatenated—into operons. This is only possible since prokaryotic ribosomes initiate translation by binding individual coding regions within the (polycistronic) mRNA. In contrast, eukaryotes initiate translation only at a single site—the 7meG "cap" structure at the 5′end of mRNA. Here, expression of proteins is achieved by the co-ordinated transcription of the individual genes located at different sites throughout the genome. The model of one gene one enzyme/one gene one polypeptide developed in the 1940s was substantially modified in the late 1960s from studies on the biogenesis of poliovirus proteins and insulin. In both these cases it was proposed proteins were formed by post-translational processing of a single precursor (poly)protein [164–167]. Encoding multiple proteins in the form of a polyprotein is a common, if not ubiquitous, strategy of viruses with positive stranded (mRNA sense) genomes. Such polyproteins are proteolytically "processed" by virus-encoded proteinases, although host-cell proteinases may also be utilised in processing virus polyproteins.

Viruses have evolved many different mechanisms to both maximise the coding capacity of their genomes and to generate multiple, different, proteins from a single ORF—many involving manipulating or modifying the host-cell translational apparatus [2]. In the case of 2A-mediated ribosome skipping, the strategy has been very widely used in biotechnology and biomedicine in the generation of transgenic cell lines/organisms as outlined above. Being able to concatenate genes in this manner has simplified and accelerated the whole process of producing transgenics: reducing, or even eliminating, the need for re-iterative rounds of transformation/selection required to introduce “traits” based upon multiple gene expression. The range of applications is immense, spanning humans, animals, plants and fungi. To conclude, the study of FMDV polyprotein processing has provided a valuable tool that has allowed researchers to create “artificial” polyproteins such that multiple, different, proteins can be generated from a single (poly)cistronic construct—driven by a single promoter. Furthermore, since 2A-mediated recoding occurs co-translationally, products can be targeted to different combinations of sub-cellular sites or secreted from the cell. Over 1500 research publications (https://www.st-andrews.ac.uk/ryan-lab/Index.html) and many patent/patent applications (https://www.freepatentonline.com/login.html) stand testament to the influence 2As have had on co-expression technology—this is not the end, this is not even the beginning of the end, this is just perhaps the end of the beginning.

Acknowledgements

The long term support of the Wellcome Trust and the Biotechnology and Biological Sciences Research Council (BBSRC) is gratefully acknowledged. The University of St Andrews is a charity registered in Scotland no. SCO13532.

Abbreviations

AAV	adeno-associated virus
BDP	bidirectional promoter
BEFV	bovine ephemeral fever virus
BHK	baby hamster kidney
BmNPV	*bombyx mori* nuclear polyhedrosis virus
BmCPV	*bombyx mori* cytoplasmic polyhedrosis virus
Bt	*Baccillus thuringiensis*
CAT	chloramphenicol acetyl-transferase
CHYSEL	*cis*-acting hydrolase element
CRISPR-Cas9	clustered regularly interspaced palindromic repeats – associated protein 9
CrPV	cricket paralysis virus
DBM	diamond back moth
DBMIV	diamondback moth iflavirus
DCV	Drosophila C virus
DERSV	duck egg-reducing syndrome virus
DNA	deoxyribonucleic acid
EoPV	*ectropis oblique* picorna-like virus
EMCV	encephalomyocarditis virus
eIFs	eukaryotic initiation factors
ER	endoplasmic reticulum
ERAV	equine rhinitis A virus
ERBV-1	equine rhinitis B virus 1
FACS	fluorescence-activated cell sorting
FMDV	foot-and-mouth disease virus

FPs	fluorescent proteins
GE	genome editing
GFP	green fluorescent protein
GR	golden rice
GUS	glucuronidase
HACKing	highly efficient and accessible system by cracking genes into the genome
HCV	hepatitis C virus
ICC	immunocytochemistry
IMNV	infectious myonecrosis virus
IP	immunoprecipitation
iPSCs	induced pluripotent stem cells
IRES	internal ribosome entry site
ITAFs	IRES trans-acting factors
mRNA	messenger RNA
NLS	nuclear localisation signal
OMRV	Omono River virus
ORF	open reading frame
OpbuCPV18	Operophtera brumata cypovirus-18
PnPV	*Perina nuda* picorna-like virus
PTV-1	porcine teschovirus-1
PV	poliovirus
RFP	red fluorescent protein
RtPV	*Rattus tanezumi* parechovirus
RNA	ribonucleic acid
SRP	signal recognition particle
TALEN	transcription activator-like effector nucleases
TaV	*Thosea asigna* virus
TCR	T-cell receptor
TEV	tobacco etch virus
TLR	Traffic Light Reporter
ToV-TJ	Tianjin totivirus
tRNA	transfer RNA
VAD	vitamin A deficiency
WP-LV	Wenzhou picorna-like virus
WCP	Wuhan carp picornavirus
YFP	yellow fluorescent protein
ZFN	zinc finger nucleases

DOI: http://dx.doi.org/10.5772/intechopen.1004928

Author details

Garry A. Luke* and Martin D. Ryan
Centre for Biomolecular Sciences, School of Biology, University of St Andrews, St Andrews, UK

*Address all correspondence to: gal@st-andrews.ac.uk

References

[1] Gesteland RF, Atkins JF. Recoding: Dynamic reprogramming of translation. Annual Review of Biochemistry. 1996;**65**:741-768

[2] Ryan MD, Luke GA. Translation of viral proteins. In: Bamford, Zuckerman M, editors. Encyclopedia of Virology. 4th ed. Vol. 1. London, New York: Elsevier; 2021. pp. 444-459. DOI:10.1016/8978-0-12-814515-9.00119-3

[3] Donnelly MLL, Luke GA, Mehrotra A, Li X, Hughes LE, Gani D, et al. Analysis of the aphthovirus 2A/2B polyprotein "cleavage" mechanism indicates not a proteolytic reaction, but a novel translational effect: A putative ribosomal "skip". Journal General Virology. 2001;**82**:1013-1025

[4] Atkins JF, Wills NM, Loughran G, Wu CY, Parsawar K, Ryan MD, et al. A case for "StopGo": reprogramming translation to augment codon meaning of GGN by promoting unconventional termination (Stop) after addition of glycine and then allowing continued translation (Go). RNA. 2007;**13**:803-810

[5] Brown JD, Ryan MD. Ribosome "skipping": "Stop-carry on" or "StopGo" translation. In: Atkins JF, Gesteland RF, editors. Recoding: Expansion of Decoding Rules Enriches Gene Expression. New York: Springer; 2010. pp. 101-122

[6] Yang X, Cheng A, Wang M, Jia R, Sun K, Pan K, et al. Structures and corresponding functions of five types of picornaviral 2A proteins. Frontiers in Microbiology. 2017;**8**:1373. DOI: 10:3389/fmicb.2017.01373

[7] Ryan MD, Belsham GJ, King AM. Specificity of enzyme-substrate interactions in foot-and-mouth disease virus polyprotein processing. Virology. 1989;**173**(1):35-45

[8] Belsham GJ. Distinctive features of the foot-and-mouth disease virus, a member of the picornavirus family; aspects of virus protein synthesis, protein processing and structure. Progress in Biophysics and Molecular Biology. 1993;**60**:241-260

[9] Ryan MD, Drew J. Foot-and-mouth disease virus 2A oligopeptide mediated cleavage of an artificial polyprotein. The EMBO Journal. 1994;**13**:928-933

[10] Sharma P, Yan F, Doronina VA, Escuin-Ordinas H, Ryan MD, Brown JD. 2A peptides provide distinct solutions to driving stop-carry on translational recoding. Nucleic Acids Research. 2012;**40**(7):3143-3151

[11] Donnelly MLL, Gani D, Flint M, Monaghan S, Ryan MD. The cleavage activities of aphthovirus and cardiovirus 2A proteins. Journal of General Virology. 1997;**78**:13-21

[12] Ryan MD, King AM, Thomas GP. Cleavage of foot-and-mouth disease virus polyprotein is mediated by residues located within a 19 amino acid sequence. Journal of General Virology. 1991;**72**:2727-2732

[13] Varshavsky A. The N-end rule. Cell. 1992;**69**(5):725-735. ISSN: 0092-8674

[14] de Felipe P, Ryan MD. Targeting of proteins derived from self-processing polyproteins containing multiple signal sequences. Traffic. 2004;**5**:616-626. DOI: 10.1111/j.1398-9219. 2004.00205.x

[15] Donnelly MLL, Hughes LE, Luke GA, Mendoza H, ten Dam E, Gani D, et al.

The "cleavage" activities of foot-and-mouth disease virus 2A site-directed mutants and naturally occurring "2A-like" sequences. Journal of General Virology. 2001;**82**:1027-1041

[16] Luke GA, de Felipe P, Lukashev A, Kallioinen SE, Bruno EA, Ryan MD. The occurrence, function, and evolutionary origins of "2A-like" sequences in virus genomes. Journal of General Virology. 2008;**89**(4):1036-1042

[17] Doronina VA, Wu C, de Felipe P, Sachs MS, Ryan MD, Brown JD. Site-specific release of nascent chains from ribosomes at a sense codon. Molecular and Cellular Biology. 2008;**28**(13):4227-4239

[18] Baranov PV, Gurvich OL, Hammer AW, Gesteland RF, Atkins JF. Recode 2003. Nucleic Acids Research. 2003;**31**:87-89

[19] Gao Z, Zhou J, Zhang J, Ding Y, Liu Y. The silent point mutations at the cleavage site of 2A/2B have no effect on the self-cleavage activity of 2A of foot-and-mouth disease virus. Infection, Genetics and Evolution. 2014;**28**:101-106

[20] Ryan MD, Donnelly MLL, Lewis A, Mehrotra AP, Wilkie J, Gani D. A model for nonstoichiometric, co-translational protein scission in eukaryotic ribosomes. Bioorganic Chemistry. 1999;**27**:55-79

[21] Kjær J, Belsham GJ. Selection of functional 2A sequences within foot-and-mouth disease virus; requirements for the NPGP motif with a distinct codon bias. RNA. 2018;**24**(1):12-17. DOI: 10.1261/rna.063339.117

[22] Hahn H, Palmenberg AC. Mutational analysis of the encephalomyocarditis virus primary cleavage. Journal Virology. 1996;**70**:6870-6875

[23] Roulston C, Luke GA, de Felipe P, Ruan L, Cope J, Nicholson J, et al. "2A-like" signal sequences mediating translational recoding: A novel form of dual protein targeting. Traffic. 2016;**17**(8):923-939

[24] Luke GA, Ryan MD. The protein coexpression problem in biotechnology and biomedicine: Virus 2A and 2A-like sequences provide a solution. Future Virology. 2013;**8**(10):983-996

[25] Novoa EM, Ribas de Pouplana L. Speeding with control: Codon usage, tRNAs, and ribosomes. Trends in Genetics. 2012;**28**:574-581

[26] Mauro VP, Chappell SA. A critical analysis of codon optimization in human therapeutics. Trends in Molecular Medicine. 2014;**20**:604-613

[27] Szymczak AL, Workman CJ, Wang Y, Vignali KM, Dilioglou S, Vanin EF, et al. Correction of multi-gene deficiency *in vivo* using a single "selfcleaving" 2A peptide-based retroviral vector. Nature Biotechnology. 2004;**22**(5):589-594

[28] Holst J, Szymczak-Workman AL, Vignali KM, Burton AR, Workman CJ, Vignali DAA. Generation of T-cell receptor retrogenic mice. Nature Protocols. 2006;**1**(1):406-417. ISSN: 1754-2189

[29] Wang X, Tian X, Marchisio MA. Logic circuits based on 2A peptide sequences in the yeast *Saccharomyces cerevisiae*. ACS Synthetic Biology. 2003;**12**:224-237

[30] Tan Y, Liang H, Chen A, Guo X. Coexpression of double or triple copies of the rabies virus glycoprotein gene using a "self-cleaving" 2A peptide-based replication-defective human adenovirus serotype 5 vector. Biologicals. 2010;**38**:586-593

[31] Yang S, Cohen CJ, Peng PD, Zhao Y, Cassard L, Yu Z, et al. Development of optimal bicistronic lentiviral vectors facilitates high-level TCR gene expression and robust tumor cell recognition. Gene Therapy. 2008;**15**(21):1411-1423

[32] Wang Y, Wang F, Wang R, Zhao P, Xia Q. 2A self-cleaving peptide-based multi-gene expression system in the silkworm *Bombyx mori*. Scientific Reports. 2015;**5**(5):16273. DOI: doi.org/10.1038/srep16273

[33] Wang Y, Wang F, Xu S, Wang R, Chen W, Hou K, et al. Optimization of a 2A self-cleaving peptide-based multigene expression system for efficient expression of upstream and downstream genes in silkworm. Molecular Genetics and Genomics. 2019;**294**(4):849-859

[34] Minskaia E, Ryan MD. Protein coexpression using FMDV 2A: Effect of "linker" residues. BioMed Research International Article. 2013;**ID 291730**. DOI: 10.1155/2013/291730

[35] Minskaia E, Nicholson J, Ryan MD. Optimisation of the foot-and-mouth disease virus 2A co-expression system for biomedical applications. BMC Biotechnology. 2013;**13**:67. Available from: http://www.biomedcentral.com/1472-6750/13/67

[36] Ho SC, Bardor M, Li B, Lee JJ, Song Z, Tong YW, et al. Comparison of internal ribosome entry site (IRES) and furin-2A (F2A) for monoclonal antibody expression level and quality in CHO cells. PLoS One. 2013;**8**:e63247

[37] Liu Z, Chen O, Wall JBJ, Zheng M, Zhou Y, Wang L, et al. Systematic comparison of 2A peptides for cloning multi-genes in a polycistronic vector. Scientific Reports. 2017;**7**:2193

[38] Subramanian V, Schuster LA, Moore KT, Taylor LE, Baker JO, Vander Wall TA, et al. A versatile 2A peptide-based bicistronic protein expressing platform for the industrial cellulase producing fungus, *Trichoderma reesei*. Biotechnology for Biofuels. 2017;**10**:34. DOI: 10.1186/s13068-017-0710-7

[39] Jiao X, Sun W, Zhang Y, Lin X, Zhang Q, Wang Q, et al. Exchanging the order of carotenogenic genes linked by porcine teschovirus-1 2A peptide enable to optimize carotenoid metabolic pathway in *Saccharomyces cerevisiae*. Royal Society of Chemistry Advances. 2018;**8**:34967

[40] Ryan MD, Luke GA, Hughes LE, Cowton VM, ten Dam E, Li X, et al. The aphtho-and cardiovirus "primary" 2A/2B polyprotein "cleavage". In: Semler BL, Wimmer E, editors. Molecular Biology of Picornaviruses. Washington DC: ASM Press; 2002. pp. 213-223

[41] Doronina VA, de Felipe P, Wu C, Sharma P, Sachs MS, Ryan MD, et al. Dissection of a co-translational nascent chain separation event. Biochemical Society Transactions. 2008;**36**(4):712-716

[42] Machida K, Mikami S, Masutani M, Mishima K, Kobayashi T, Imataka H. A translation system reconstituted with human factors proves that processing of encephalomyocarditis virus proteins 2A and 2B occurs in the elongation phase of translation without eukaryotic release factors. Journal of Biological Chemistry. 2014;**289**(46):31960-31971

[43] Kim JH, Lee SR, Li L-H, Park H-J, Park J-H, Lee KY, et al. High cleavage efficiency of a 2A peptide derived from porcine teschovirus-1 in human cell lines, zebrafish and mice. PLOS One. 2011;**6**(4):e18556. DOI: 10.1371/journal.pone.0018556

[44] Chng J, Wang T, Nian R, Lau A, Hoi KM, Ho SC, et al. Cleavage efficient 2A peptides for high level

monoclonal antibody expression in CHO cells. MAbs. 2015;**7**:403-412. DOI: 10.1080/19420862.2015.1008351

[45] Zhu X, Ricci-Tam C, Hager ER, Sgro AE. Self-cleaving 2A peptides for expression of multiple genes in *Dictyostelium discoideum*. PLoS One. 2023;**18**(3). DOI: 10.1371/journal.pone.0281211

[46] de Felipe P, Hughes LE, Ryan MD, Brown JD. Co-translational, intraribosomal cleavage of polypeptides by the foot-and-mouth disease virus 2A peptide. The Journal of Biological Chemistry. 2003;**13**:11441-11448

[47] Geier M, Fauland P, Vogl T, Glieder A. Compact multi-enzyme pathways in *P. pastoris*. Chemical Communications. 2015;**51**:1643-1646

[48] Souza-Moreira TM, Navarrete C, Chen X, Zanelli CF, Valentini SR, Furlan M, et al. Screening of 2A peptides for polycistronic gene expression in yeast. FEMS Yeast Research. 2018;**18**(5). DOI: 10.1093/femsyr/foy036

[49] Hoefgen S, Lin J, Fricke J, Stroe MC, Mattern DJ, Kufs JE, et al. Facile assembly and fluorescence-based screening method for heterologous expression of biosynthetic pathways in fungi. Metabolic Engineering. 2018;**48**:44-51

[50] Rasala BA, Chao S-S, Pier M, Barrera DJ, Mayfield SP. Enhanced genetic tools for engineering multigene traits into green algae. PLoS One. 2014;**9**(4):e94028. DOI: 10.1371/journal.pone.0094028

[51] Koh HG, Kang NK, Kim EK, Jeon S, Shin S-E, Lee B, et al. Advanced multigene expression system for *Nannochloropsis Salina* using 2A self-cleaning peptides. Journal of Biotechnology. 2018;**278**:39-47

[52] Burén S, Ortega-Villasante C, Ötvös K, Samuelsson G, Bakó L, Villarejo A. Use of the foot-and-mouth disease virus 2A peptide co-expression system to study intracellular protein trafficking in Arabidopsis. PLoS One. 2012;**7**(12):eS1973. DOI: 10.1371/journal.pone.0051973

[53] Zhang B, Rapolu M, Kumar S, Gupta M, Liang Z, Han Z, et al. Coordinated protein co-expression in plants by harnessing the synergy between an intein and a viral 2A peptide. Plant Biotechnology Journal. 2017;**15**:718-728. DOI: 10.1111/pbi.12670

[54] Provost E, Rhee J, Leach SD. Viral 2A peptides allow expression of multiple proteins from a single ORF in transgenic zebrafish embryos. Genesis. 2007;**45**(10):625-629

[55] Jeong I, Kim E, Seong JY, Park HC. Overexpression of Spexin 1 in the dorsal habenula reduced anxiety in zebrafish. Frontiers in Neural Circuits. 2019;**13**:1-8. DOI: doi.org/10.3389/fncir2019.00053

[56] Grabert K, Sehgal A, Irvine KM, Wollscheid-Lengeling E, Ozdemir DD, Stables J, et al. A transgenic line that reports CSFIR protein expression provides a definitive marker for the mouse mononuclear phagocyte system. The Journal of Immunology. 2020;**205**(11):3154-3166. DOI: 10.4049/jimmunol.2000835

[57] El Amrani A, Barakate A, Askari BM, Li X, Roberts AG, Ryan MD, et al. Coordinate expression and independent subcellular targeting of multiple proteins from a single transgene. Plant Physiology. 2004;**135**:16-24

[58] Yan J, Wang H, Xu Q, Jain N, Toxavidis V, Tigges J, et al. Signal sequence is still required in genes downstream of "autocleaving" 2A

peptide for secretary or membrane-anchored expression. Analytical Biochemistry. 2010;**399**:144-146

[59] Trichas G, Begbie J, Srinivas S. Use of the viral 2A peptide for bicistronic expression in transgenic mice. BioMed Central BMC Biology. 2008;**6**:40. ISSN: 1741-7007

[60] Kumagai H, Matsuura T, Kato Y, Watanabe H. Development of a bicistronic expression system in the branchiopod crustacean *Daphnia magna*. Genesis. 2017;**55**:e23083. DOI: 10.1002/dvg.23083

[61] Mukherjee M, Wang ZQ. A well-characterized polycistronic-like gene expression system in yeast. Biotechnology and Bioengineering. 2023;**120**:260-271

[62] Fang J, Qian JJ, Yi S, Harding TC, Tu GH, VanRoey M, et al. Stable antibody expression at therapeutic levels using the 2A peptide. Nature Biotechnology. 2005;**23**(5):584-590

[63] François IEJA, van Hemelrijck W, Aerts AM, Wouters PFJ, Proost P, Broekaert WF, et al. Processing in *Arabidopsis thaliana* of a heterologous polyprotein resulting in differential targeting of the individual plant defensins. Plant Science. 2004;**166**:113-121. ISSN: 0168-9452

[64] Mizote Y, Masumi-Koizumi K, Katsuda T, Yamaji H. Production of an antibody fab fragment using 2A peptide in insect cells. Journal of Bioscience and Bioengineering. 2020;**130**(2):205-211

[65] Lo Y-T, Tulloch F, Wu H-C, Luke GA, Ryan MD, Chu C-Y. Expression and immunogenicity of secreted forms of bovine ephemeral fever virus glycoproteins applied to subunit vaccine development. Journal of Applied Microbiology. 2021;**131**(3):1123-1135. DOI: 10.1111/jam.15044

[66] Lo Y-T, Ryan MD, Luke GA, Chang W-C, Wu H-C. Immunogenicity of a secreted, C-terminally truncated, form of bovine viral diarrhea virus E2 glycoprotein as a potential candidate in subunit vaccine development. Scientific Reports. 2023;**13**:296. DOI: 10.1038/s41598-022-26766-y

[67] de Felipe P, Luke GA, Hughes LE, Gani D, Halpin C, Ryan MD. *E unum pluribus:* Multiple proteins from a self-processing polyprotein. Trends in Biotechnology. 2006;**24**(2):68-75. ISSN: 0167-7799

[68] de Felipe P, Luke GA, Brown JD, Ryan MD. Inhibition of 2A-mediated "cleavage" of certain artificial polyproteins bearing N-terminal signal sequences. Biotechnology Journal. 2010;**5**(2):213-223. ISSN: 1860-6768

[69] Lengler J, Holzmüller H, Salmons B, Günzburg WH, Renner M. FMDV – 2A sequence and protein arrangement contribute to functionality of CYP2B1–reporter fusion protein. Analytical Biochemistry. 2005;**343**:116-124. DOI: 10.1016/j.ab.2005.05.004

[70] Rothwell DG, Crossley R, Bridgeman JS, Sheard V, Zhang Y, Sharp TV, et al. Functional expression of secreted proteins from a bicistronic retroviral cassette based on foot-and-mouth disease virus 2A can be position dependent. Human Gene Therapy. 2010;**21**:1631-1637. DOI: 10.1089/hum.2009.197

[71] Reinhardt A, Kagawa H, Woltjen K. N-terminal amino acids determine KL4F protein stability in 2A peptide-linked polycistronic reprogramming constructs. Stem Cell Reports. 2020;**14**:520-527. DOI: 10.1016/j.stemcr.2020.01.014

[72] de Lima JGS, Lanza DCF. 2A and 2A-like sequences: Distribution in different virus species and applications in biotechnology. Viruses. 2021;**13**:2160. DOI: 10.3390/v13112160

[73] de Lima JGS, Teixeira DG, Freitas TT, Lima JPMS, Lanza DCF. Evolutionary origin of 2A-like sequences in *Totiviridae* genomes. Virus Research. 2019;**259**:1-9

[74] Su X, Shuo D, Luo Y, Pan X, Yan D, Li X, et al. An emerging duck egg-reducing syndrome caused by a novel picornavirus containing seven putative 2A peptides. Viruses. 2022;**14**:932. DOI: 10.3390/v14050932

[75] Heras SR, Thomas MC, García-Canadas M, de Felipe P, García-Perez JL, Ryan MD, et al. L1Tc non-LTR retrotransposons from *Trypanosoma cruzi* contain a functional viral-like self-cleaving 2A sequence in frame with the active proteins they encode. Cellular and Molecular Life Sciences. 2006;**63**:1449-1460

[76] Odon V, Luke GA, Roulston C, de Felipe P, Ruan L, Escuin-Ordinas H, et al. APE-type non-LTR retrotransposons of multicellular organisms encode virus-like 2A oligopeptide sequences, which mediate translational recoding during protein synthesis. Molecular Biology and Evolution. 2013;**30**(8):1955-1965

[77] Luke GA, Pathania US, Roulston C, de Felipe P, Ryan MD. DxExNPGP – Motives for the motif. Recent Research Developments in Virology. 2014;**9**:25-42

[78] Sun WW, Zhang B, Han Z, Kumar S, Gupta M. Non-viral 2A-like sequences for protein coexpression. Journal of Biotechnology. 2022;**358**:1-8

[79] Osborn MJ, Panoskaltsis-Mortari A, McElmurry RT, Bell SK, Vignali DAA, Ryan MD, et al. A picornaviral 2A-like sequence-based tricistronic vector allowing for high-level therapeutic gene expression coupled to a dual-reporter system. Molecular Therapy. 2005;**12**:569-574

[80] Daniels RW, Rossano AJ, Macleod GT, Ganetzky B. Expression of multiple transgenes from a single construct using viral 2A peptides in *Drosophila*. PLoS One. 2014;**9**(6):e100637. DOI: 10.1371/journal.pone.0100637

[81] Diao F, White BH. A novel approach for directing transgene expression in *Drosophila*: T2A–Gal4 in-frame fusion. Genetics. 2012;**190**:1139-1144

[82] Efimova VS, Isaeva LV, Orekhov PS, Bozdaganyan ME, Rubtsov MA, Novikova LA. Using a viral 2A peptide-based strategy to reconstruct the bovine P450scc steroidogenic system in *S. cerevisiae*. Bovine P450scc system expression using 2A peptides. Journal of Biotechnology. 2021;**325**:186-195

[83] Yue Q, Meng J, Qiu Y, Yin M, Zhang L, Zhou W, et al. A polycistronic system for multiplexed and precalibrated expression of multigene pathways in fungi. Nature Communications. 2023;**14**:4267. DOI: 10.1038/s41467-023-40027 0

[84] Pelletier J, Sonenberg N. Internal initiation of translation of eukaryotic mRNA directed by a sequence derived from poliovirus RNA. Nature. 1988;**334**:320-325

[85] Jang SK, Krausslich HG, Nicklin MJ, Duke GM, Palmenberg AC, Wimmer E. A segment of the 5′ nontranslated region of encephalomycarditis virus RNA detects internal entry of ribosomes during *in vitro* translation. Journal Virology. 1988;**62**(8):2636-2643

[86] Bieleski L, Talbot S. Kaposi's sarcoma-associated herpesvirus vCyclin

open reading frame contains an internal ribosome entry site. Journal Virology. 2001;**75**:1864-1869

[87] Tahiri-Alaoui A, Smith LP, Baigent S, Kgosana L, Petherbridge LJ, Lambeth LS, et al. Identification of an intercistronic internal ribosome entry site in a Marek's disease virus immediate-early gene. Journal Virology. 2009;**83**:5846-5853

[88] Jackson RJ, Hellen CU, Pestova TV. The mechanism of eukaryotic translation initiation and principles of its regulation. Nature Reviews Molecular Cell Biology. 2010;**11**:113-127

[89] Hinnebusch AG. The scanning mechanism of eukaryotic translation initiation. Annual Review of Biochemistry. 2014;**83**:779-812. DOI: 10.1146/annurev-biochem-060713-035802

[90] Yamamoto H, Unbehaun A, Spahn CMT. Ribosomal chamber music toward an understanding of IRES mechanisms. Trends in Biochemical Sciences. 2017;**42**:655-668. DOI: 10.1016/j.tibs2017.06.002

[91] Godet AC, David F, Hantelys F, Tatin F, Lacazette E, Garmy-Susini B, et al. IRES trans-acting factors, key actors of the stress response. International Journal of Molecular Science. 2019;**20**(4):924. DOI: 10.3390/ijms20040924

[92] Jan E, Mohr I, Walsh D. A Cap-to-Tail guide to mRNA translation strategies in virus-infected cells. Annual Review of Virology. 2016;**3**:283-307. DOI: 10.1146/annurev-virology.100114-055014

[93] Jaafar ZA, Kieft JS. Viral RNA structure-based strategies to manipulate translation. Nature Reviews Microbiology. 2019;**17**:110-123. DOI: 10.1038/s41579-018-0117-x

[94] Filbin ME, Kieft JS. Toward a structural understanding of IRES RNA function. Current Opinions in Structural Biology. 2009;**19**:267-276. DOI: 10.1016/sbi.2009.03.005

[95] Johnson AG, Grosely R, Petrov AN, Puglisi JD. Dynamics of IRES-mediated translation. Philosophical Transactions of the Royal Society B: Biological Sciences. 2017;**372**:20160177. DOI: 10.1098/rstb.2016.0177

[96] Borman AM, Bailly JL, Girard M, Kean KM. Picornavirus internal ribosome entry segments: Comparison of translation efficiency and the requirements for optimal internal initiation of translation *in vitro*. Nucleic Acids Research. 1995;**23**:3656-3663

[97] Borman AM, Le Mercier P, Girard M, Kean KM. Comparison of picornaviral-IRES driven internal initiation of translation in cultured cells of different origins. Nucleic Acids Research. 1997;**25**:925-932

[98] Oumard A, Hennecke M, Hauser H, Nourbakhsh M. Translation of NRF mRNA is mediated by highly efficient internal ribosome entry. Molecular and Cellular Biology. 2000;**20**:2755-2759

[99] Dirks W, Wirth M, Hauser H. Bicistronic transcription units for gene expression in mammalian cells. Gene. 1993;**128**:247-249

[100] Müller P, Oumard A, Wirth D, Kröger A, Hauser H. Polyvalent vectors for coexpression of multiple genes. In: Schleef M, editor. Plasmids for Therapy and Vaccination. Weinheim, Germany: Wiley-VCH; 2001. pp. 119-137

[101] Hellen C, Sarnow P. Internal ribosome entry sites in eukaryotic mRNA molecules. Genes and Development. 2001;**15**:1593-1612

[102] Mizuguchi H, Xu Z, Ishii-Watabe A, Uchida E, Hayakawa T. IRES-dependent second gene expression is significantly lower than cap-dependent first gene expression in a bicistronic vector. Molecular Therapy. 2000;**1**:376-382. ISSN: 1525-0016

[103] Martin P, Albagli O, Poggi MC, Boulukos KE, Pognonec P. Development of a new bicistronic retroviral vector with strong IRES activity. BMC Biotechnology. 2006;**6**:4

[104] Ha S-H, Liang YS, Jung H, Ahn M-J, Suh S-C, Kweon S-J, et al. Application of two bicistronic systems involving 2A and IRES sequences to the biosynthesis of carotenoids in rice endosperm. Plant Biotechnology Journal. 2010;**8**:928-938. ISSN: 1467-7644

[105] Douin V, Bornes S, Creancier L, Rochaix P, Favre G, Prats AC, et al. Use and comparison of different internal ribosome entry sites (IRES) in tricistronic retroviral vectors. BMC Biotechnology. 2004;**4**:16. DOI: 10.1186/1472-6750-4-16

[106] Renaud-Gabardos E, Hantelys F, Morfoisse F, Chaufour X, Garmy-Susini B, Prats AC. Internal ribosome entry site-based vectors for combined gene therapy. World Journal of Experimental Medicine. 2015;**5**(1):11-20. ISSN: 2220-315X

[107] Urwin P, Zubko E, Atkinson H. The biotechnological application and limitation of IRES to deliver multiple defence genes to plant pathogens. Physiological and Molecular Plant Pathology. 2002;**61**:103-108

[108] El-Banna A, Hajiezaei MR, Wissing J, Ali Z, Vass L. Over-expression of PR-10a leads to increased salt and osmotic tolerance in potato cell cultures. Journal of Biotechnology. 2010;**150**:277-287

[109] Garanina EE, Mukhamedshina YO, Salafutdinov II, Kiyasov AP, Lima LM, Reis HJ, et al. Construction of recombinant adenovirus containing picorna-viral 2A-peptide sequence for the co-expression of neuro-protective growth factors in human umbilical cord blood cells. Spinal Cord. 2016;**54**:423-430

[110] Lewis JE, Brameld JM, Hill P, Barrett P, Ebling FJP, Jethwa PH. The use of a viral 2A sequence for the simultaneous over-expression of both the vgf gene and enhanced green fluorescent protein (eGFP) *in vitro* and *in vivo*. Journal of Neuroscience Methods. 2015;**256**:22-29

[111] Browne EP. An interleukin-1 beta-encoding retrovirus exhibits enhanced replication *in vivo*. Journal of Virology. 2015;**89**:155-164

[112] Peng Y, Yang T, Tang X, Chen F, Wang S. Construction of an inducible CRISPR/Cas9 system for CXCR4 gene and demonstration of its effects on MKN-45 cells. Cell Biochemistry and Biophysics. 2020;**78**:23-30

[113] Luke GA. Translating 2A research into practice. In: Agbo EC, editor. Innovations in Biotechnology. Croatia: InTech; 2012. pp. 161-186. DOI: 10.5772/30091

[114] Luke GA, Roulston C, Tilsner J, Ryan MD. Growing uses of 2A in plant biotechnology. In: D Ekinci editor. Biotechnology. Croatia: InTech; 2015. p. 165-193. DOI: 10.5772/59878

[115] Luke GA, Ryan MD. Therapeutic applications of the "NPGP" family of viral 2As. Reviews in Medical Virology. 2018;**28**(6):1-12. DOI: 10.1002/rmv.2001

[116] Schwarzhans J-P, Luttermann T, Geier M, Kalinowski J, Friehs K. Towards systems metabolic engineering in *Pichia*

pastoris. Biotechnology Advances. 2017;**35**:681-710

[117] Tian Y, Li Y, Zhao F, Meng C. Engineered *Pichia pastoris* production of fusaruside, a selective immunomodulator. BMC Biotechnology. 2019;**19**:37. DOI: 10.1186/s12896-019-0532-8

[118] Karbalaei M, Rezaee SA, Farsiani H. *Pichia pastoris*: A highly successful expression system for optimal synthesis of heterologous proteins. Journal of Cell Physiology. 2020;**235**(9):5867-5881

[119] Zulfiqar F, Ashraf M, Siddique KHM. Role of glycine betaine in the thermotolerance of plants. Agronomy. 2022;**12**:276. DOI: 10.3390/agronomy1202027

[120] Wang S, Yao Q, Tao J, Qiao Y, Zhang Z. Co-ordinate expression of glycine betaine synthesis genes linked by the FMDV 2A region in a single open reading frame in *Pichia pastoris*. Applied Microbiology Biotechnology. 2007;**77**:891-899

[121] Siripong W, Wolf P, Kusumoputri TP, Downes JJ, Kocharin K, Tanapongpipat S, et al. Metabolic engineering of *Pichia pastoris* for production of isobutanol and isobutyl acetate. Biotechnology for Biofuels. 2018;**11**:1. DOI: 10.1186/s13068-017-1003-x

[122] Siripong W, Angela C, Tanapongpipat S, Runguphan W. Metabolic engineering of *Pichia pastoris* for production of isopentanol (3-Methyl-1-butanol). Enzyme and Microbial Technology. 2020;**138**:109557. DOI: 10.1016/j.enzmictec.2020.109557

[123] Park M, Kang K, Park S, Kim YS, Ha S-H, Lee SW, et al. Expression of serotonin derivative synthetic genes on a single self-processing polypeptide and the production of serotonin derivatives in microbes. Applied Microbiology and Biotechnology. 2008;**81**:43-49

[124] Cruz-Teran CA, Tiruthani K, Mischler A, Rao BM. Inefficient ribosomal skipping enables simultaneous secretion and display of proteins in *Saccharomyces cerevisiae*. ACS Synthetic Biology. 2017;**6**:2096-2107

[125] Verba KA, Agard DA. Protein expression and purification of the Hsp90-Cdc37-Cdk4 kinase complex from *Saccharomyces cerevisiae*. Bio-Protocol. 2017;**7**(19):e2563

[126] Grzeschik J, Hinz SC, Könning D, Pirzer T, Becker S, Zielonka S, et al. A simplified procedure for antibody engineering by yeast surface display: Coupling display levels and target binding by ribosomal skipping. Biotechnology Journal. 2017;**12**(2). DOI: 10.1002/biot.201600454

[127] Rosowski S, Becker S, Toleikis L, Valldorf B, Grzeschik J, Demir D, et al. A novel one-step approach for the construction of yeast surface display fab antibody libraries. Microbial Cell Factories. 2018;**17**(1):3

[128] Botman D, de Groot DH, Schmidt P, Goedhart J, Teusink B. *In vivo* characterisation of fluorescent proteins in budding yeast. Scientific Reports. 2019;**9**(1):2234

[129] Brazier-Hicks M, Edwards R. Metabolic engineering of the flavone-C-glycoside pathway using polyprotein technology. Metabolic Engineering. 2013;**16**:11-20

[130] Beekwilder J, van Rossom HM, Koopman F, Sonntag F, Buchhaupt M, Schrader J, et al. Polycistronic expression of β-carotene biosynthetic pathway

in *Saccharomyces cerevisiae* coupled to β-ionone production. Journal of Biotechnology. 2014;**192**:383-392

[131] Rajput R, Naik J, Misra P, Trivedi PK, Pandey A. Gene pyramiding in transgenic plant development: Approaches and challenges. Journal of Plant Growth Regulation. 2023;**42**:6038-6056. DOI: 10.1007/s00344-022-10760-9

[132] Randall J, Sutton D, Ghoshroy S, Bagga S, Kemp JD. Co-ordinate expression of β- and δ- zeins in transgenic tobacco. Plant Science. 2004;**167**:367-372

[133] Quilis J, López-García B, Meynard D, Guiderdoni E, Segundo BS. Inducible expression of a fusion gene encoding two proteinase inhibitors leads to insect and pathogen resistance in transgenic rice. Plant Biotechnology Journal. 2014;**12**:367-377

[134] Zhao Q, Liu M, Tan M, Gao J, Shen Z. Expression of Cry1Ab and Cry2Ab by a polycistronic transgene with a self-cleavage peptide in rice. PLoS One. 2014;**9**(10):e10006. DOI: 10.1371/journal.pone.0110006

[135] Liu X, Yang W, Mu B, Li S, Zhou X, Zhang C, et al. Engineering of "Purple Embryo Maize" with a multigene expression system derived from a bidirectional promoter and self-cleaving 2A peptides. Plant Biotechnology Journal. 2018;**16**:1107-1109

[136] Ye X, Al-Babili S, Klöti A, Zhang J, Lucca P, Beyer P, et al. Engineering the provitamin A (beta-carotene) biosynthetic pathway into (carotenoid-free rice) endosperm. Science. 2000;**287**(5451):303-305. DOI: 10.1126/science.287.5451.303

[137] Paine JA, Shipton CA, Chaggar S, Howells RM, Kennedy MJ, Vernon G, et al. Improving the nutritional value of golden rice through increased pro-vitamin A content. Nature Biotechnology. 2005;**23**:482-487

[138] Jeong YS, Ku H-K, Kim JK, You MK, Lim S-H, Kim J-K, et al. Effect of codon optimization on the enhancement of the β-carotene contents in rice endosperm. Plant Biotechnology Reports. 2017;**11**:171-179

[139] Kim M-J, Kim JK, Kim HJ, Pak JH, Lee J-H, Kim D-H, et al. Genetic modification of the soybean to enhance the β-carotene content through seed-specific expression. PLoS One. 2012;**7**(10):e48287. DOI: 10.1371/journal.pone.0048287

[140] Saini RK, Keum Y-S, Daglia M, Rengasamy KRR. Dietary carotenoids in cancer chemoprevention and chemotherapy: A review of emerging evidence. Pharmacological Research. 2020;**157**:104830

[141] Ralley L, Enfissi EMA, Misawa N, Schuch W, Bramley PM, Fraser PD. Metabolic engineering of ketocarotenoid formation in higher plants. The Plant Journal. 2004;**39**:477-486

[142] Zhu C, Zhu C, Naqvi S, Capell T, Christou P. Metabolic engineering of ketocarotenoid biosynthesis in higher plants. Archives of Biochemistry and Biophysics. 2009;**483**:182-190

[143] Ha S-H, Kim JK, Jeong YS, You M-K, Lim S-H, Kim J-K. Stepwise pathway engineering to the biosynthesis of zeaxanthin, astaxanthin and capsanthin in rice endosperm. Metabolic Engineering. 2019;**52**:178-189

[144] Jeong YS, Ku H-K, Jung Y-J, Kim JK, Lee KB, Kim J-K, et al. 2A-linked bi-, tri-, and quad-cistrons for the stepwise biosynthesis of β-carotene, zeaxanthin, and ketocarotenoids in rice endosperm.

Metabolic Engineering Communications. 2021;**12**:e00166

[145] Unkles SE, Valiante V, Mattern DJ, Brakhage AA. Synthetic biology tools for bioprospecting of natural products in eukaryotes. Chemistry & Biology. 2014;**21**:502-508

[146] Samalova M, Fricker M, Moore I. Ratio-metric fluorescence-imaging assays of plant membrane traffic using polyproteins. Traffic. 2006;7:1701-1723

[147] Ding Q, Lee YK, Schaefer EA, Peters DT, Veres A, Kim K, et al. A TALEN genome-editing system for generating human stem cell-based disease models. Cell Stem Cell. 2013;**12**(2):238-251. DOI: 10.1016/j.stem.2012.11.011

[148] Duda K, Lonowski LA, Kofoed-Nielsen M, Ibarra A, Delay CM, Kang Q, et al. High-efficiency genome editing *via* 2A-coupled co-expression of fluorescent proteins and zinc finger nucleases or CRISPR/Cas9 nickase pairs. Nucleic Acids Research. 2014;**42**(10):e84. DOI: 10.1093/nar/gku251

[149] Kim H, Kim M-S, Wee G. Magnetic separation and antibiotics selection enable enrichment of cells with ZFN/TALEN-induced mutations. PLoSONE. 2013;**8**(2):e56476. DOI: 10.1371/journa.pne.0056476

[150] Certo MT, Ryu BY, Annis JE, Garibov M, Jarjour J, Rawlings DJ, et al. Tracking genome engineering outcome at individual DNA breakpoints. Nature Methods. 2011;**8**(8):671-676

[151] Moore R, Spinhirne A, Lai MJ, Preisser S, Li Y, Kang T, et al. CRISPR-based self-cleaving mechanism for controllable gene delivery in human cells. Nucleic Acids Research. 2015;**43**(2):1297-1303. DOI: 10.1093/nar/gku1326

[152] Hofmann A, Falk J, Prangemeier T, Happel D, Köber A, Christmann A, et al. A tightly regulated and adjustable CRISPR-dCas9 based AND gate in yeast. Nucleic Acids Research. 2019;**47**(1):509-520. DOI: 10.1093/nar/gky1191

[153] Nakamura M, Srinivasan P, Chavez M, Carter MA, Dominguez AA, La Russa M, et al. Anti-CRISPR-mediated control of gene editing and synthetic circuits in eukaryotic cells. Nature Communications. 2019;**10**(1):194. DOI: 10.1038/s41467-018-08158x

[154] Arevalo-Villalobos JI, Govea-Alonso DO, Bañuelos-Hernández B, González-Ortega O, Zarazúa S, Rosales-Mendoza S. Inducible expression of antigens in plants: A study focused on peptides related to multiple sclerosis immunotherapy. Journal of Biotechnology. 2020;**318**:51-56

[155] Lin Y, Hu CC, Liao JT, Lee YL, Huang YW, Lin NS, et al. An effective way of producing fully assembled antibody in transgenic tobacco plants by linking heavy and light chains *via* a self-cleaving 2A peptide. Frontiers in Plant Science. 2018;**9**:1-11

[156] Walker PJ, Klement E. Epidemiology and control of bovine ephemeral fever. Veterinary Research. 2015;**46**:124. DOI: 10.1186/s13567-015-0262-4

[157] Walker PJ, Byrne KA, Cybinski DH, Doolan DL, Wang Y. Proteins of bovine ephemeral fever virus. Journal of General Virology. 1991;**72**:67-74

[158] Almasi S, Bakhshesh M. Antigenic variation of bovine ephemeral fever viruses isolated in Iran, 2012-2013. Virus Genes. 2019;**55**:654-659. DOI: 10.1007/s11262-019-01688-6

[159] Richter V, Lebl K, Baumgartner W, Obritzhauser W, Käsbohrer A, Pinior B. A systematic worldwide review of the

direct monetary losses in cattle due to bovine viral diarrhoea virus infection. The Veterinary Journal. 2017;**220**:80-87. DOI: 10.1016/j.tvjl.2017.01.005

[160] Donis RO, Corapi W, Dubovi EJ. Neutralizing monoclonal antibodies to bovine viral diarrhoea virus bind to the 56K and 58K glycoprotein. Journal of General Virology. 1988;**69**:77-86

[161] Park K, Jeong J, Chung BH. Live imaging of cellular dynamics using a multi-imaging vector in single cells. Chemical Communications. 2014;**50**:10734

[162] Jeyarajan S, Zhang IX, Arvan P, Lentz SI, Satin LS. Simultaneous measurement of changes in mitochondrial and endoplasmic reticulum free calcium in pancreatic beta cells. Biosensors. 2023;**13**:382. DOI: 10.3390/bios13030382

[163] Schwirz J, Yan Y, Franta Z, Schetelig MF. Bicistronic expression and differential localization of proteins in insect cells and *Drosophila suzukii* using picornaviral 2A peptides. Insect Biochemistry and Molecular Biology. 2020;**119**.103324

[164] Summers DF, Maizel JV. Evidence for large precursor proteins in poliovirus synthesis. Proceedings of the National Academy of Sciences USA. 1968;**59**:966-971. DOI: 10.1073/pnas.59.3.966

[165] Grant PT, Reid KB. Biosynthesis of an insulin precursor by cod islet tissue and the occurrence of intermediates in the conversion to insulin. Biochemical Journal. 1968;**109**(3):32P. DOI: 10.1042/bj1090032pa

[166] Chance RE, Ellis RM, Bromer WW. Porcine proinsulin: Characterization and amino acid sequence. Science. 1968;**161**(3837):165-167. DOI: 10.1126/science.161.3837.165

[167] Tung AK, Yip CC. The biosynthesis of insulin and "proinsulin" in foetal bovine pancreas. Diabetologia. 1968;**4**:68-70